Medicine on the Periphery

Medicine on the Periphery

Public Health in Yucatán, Mexico, 1870–1960

David Sowell

LEXINGTON BOOKS
Lanham • Boulder • New York • London

Published by Lexington Books
An imprint of The Rowman & Littlefield Publishing Group, Inc.
4501 Forbes Boulevard, Suite 200, Lanham, Maryland 20706
www.rowman.com

Unit A, Whitacre Mews, 26-34 Stannary Street, London SE11 4AB

British Library Cataloguing in Publication Information Available

Library of Congress Cataloging-in-Publication Data
Sowell, David, 1952– , author.
Medicine on the periphery : public health in the Yucatan, Mexico, 1870-1960 / David Sowell.
p. ; cm.
Includes bibliographical references and index.
ISBN 978-1-4985-1734-8 (cloth : alk. paper) — ISBN 978-1-4985-1735-5 (electronic)
[DNLM: 1. Public Health—history—Mexico. 2. Delivery of Health Care—history—Mexico. 3. History, 19th Century—Mexico. 4. History, 20th Century—Mexico. 5. Politics—Mexico. 6. Social Environment—Mexico. WA 11 DM4] I. Title.
RA395.M6
362.10972—dc23 2015033422

♾™ The paper used in this publication meets the minimum requirements of American National Standard for Information Sciences—Permanence of Paper for Printed Library Materials, ANSI/NISO Z39.48-1992.

Printed in the United States of America

For Chris

With eternal gratitude for the formation of "Sowell Inc."

Contents

Preface

Where were the conflicts?

I had come to Mérida to investigate social and ethnic tensions associated with changes in the practice of medicine and public health in Yucatán, Mexico. Like many students of my generation, Robert Redfield and Nelson Reed had provided a fascinating introduction to Yucatán. Both scholars stressed conflict between Maya peoples and forces of modernization as central to the history of the region. Reed had offered a compelling account of the mid-nineteenth-century "Caste War" that pitted rural Maya peoples against white Mexicans concentrated in the urban centers of Valladolid and Mérida.[1] Redfield had formulated a social vision of Yucatán that ranged from the "traditional" peoples of Quintana Roo to the rapidly changing lifestyles of twentieth-century Mérida.[2] My earlier research in Colombia and Ecuador had suggested that the introduction of biomedicine—a medical system that viewed the body as a biological machine that responded to "natural" forces—would produce diverse social dislocations as traditional norms encountered forces of "modernization."[3] I expected, for example, that Maya healers would come into frequent conflict with biomedical practitioners, and that Mexicans with deep Catholic beliefs would find the biomedical emphasis upon secular natural authority sacrilegious and threatening. (Terms such as biomedicine are discussed below.)

This hypothesis rapidly collapsed within a few weeks of research in the inviting *Archivo General del Estado de Yucatán* (AGEY) in Mérida. Juridical files revealed a few minor cases and records of the *Junta Superior de Sanidad* (General Board of Health) suggested some instances of traditional healers practicing without an academic title, but no significant patterns of conflict were visible. Investigations in Mexico City in the *Archivo General de la Nación* (AGN) and the *Archivo Histórico de la Secretaría de Salubridad y Asistencia* (AHSSA) also failed to produce evidence of social conflict surrounding biomedicalization, though they did reveal substantive tensions between public health officials in Mérida and in the Mexican capital.

The overwhelming sense from archival materials was of the development of an extensive public health organization in Yucatán and the gradual expansion of biomedical institutions from Mérida into the "interior" of the state. This was especially visible in the 217 volumes of the *Copiador de Oficios*, a synopsis of daily activities of the *Junta Superior* that spanned the 1890s through the 1940s. The character of public health appeared to change in the 1930s, as the revolutionary regime of Lázaro Cárdenas (1934–1940) brought new priorities to the region. A quick survey of materials at the AGEY and at the *La Hemeroteca del Estado "José María Pino Suárez"* in the *Biblioteca Yucatanse* offered evidence of an extensive medical press, at times associated with the *Junta Superior*, but more often with medical associations. Notable was the *Revista Médica de Yucatán*, published by the *Sociedad Médica Yucateca* (Yucatec Medical Society, SMY) from 1906 until 1955. Archival materials generally shape the trajectory of investigations; mine was toward an institutional history of public health in Yucatán that sustained the biomedicalization of the state.

Archives in Mérida and Mexico City offer distinct insights into the history of public health in Yucatán. Medical practitioners and public health officers in both cities held similar understandings of the importance of biomedicine to a modernizing nation. Their attitudes differed however, in that leaders in Yucatán stressed local activities, while federal perspectives came to encompass the entire nation. Initially, federal jurisdiction over public health matters was limited by the Constitution of 1857 to questions of communicable diseases at ports and frontiers. This left Yucatec officials with functional autonomy over the development of public health in the region, a process evident in the records of the *Junta Superior de Sanidad*. In the wake of the Revolution however, national officials sought to recast the jurisdiction of the federal *Departamento de Salubridad Pública* (Department of Public Health, DSP) to subordinate state and local officials to the authority of Mexico City. Federal attention to Yucatán increased dramatically with the Cárdenas regime, forcing Yucatec officials to create health care programs on the newly nationalized henequen *ejidos* (collectively owned estates). Simmering tensions seemed omnipresent between Mérida and Mexico City. Yucatec records tend to reflect the primacy of state efforts; federal archives tend to reveal the efforts of officials sought to shape Yucatec health programs in keeping with revolutionary objectives. The project clearly had to pay close attention to the often troubled relationship between the state and federal governments.

The tensions between Yucatán and Mexico visible in the archives are echoed in the central plaza in contemporary Mérida. In shops bordering the plaza, one can buy images of the flag that the Republic of Yucatán flew during its brief separation from Mexico in the 1840s, reflecting a strong sense of Yucatec "nationalism." The architecture around the plaza suggests the complexity of the region's history. The conquest imagery of the conqueror Francisco Montejo parallels that of the cathedral, both of which are constructed from stone from the indigenous city of T'hó upon which Mérida was built. The symbolism of colonial power over indigenous populations cannot be clearer. The Peón Contreras Theater (1912) speaks to the grandeur of the age of henequen, when the economic and political elite supported the modernization of the capital, including the showpiece *Paseo Montejo* just to the north of the city center. Another image of Yucatán is conveyed in the murals of Fernando Castro Pacheco in the Governor's Palace, which exalts Maya resistance to Spanish rule and the brutality of labor under the henequen regime.

Whether one glorifies or vilifies the age of henequen, the economic history of Yucatán during the henequen era (ca. 1870–1950) is critically important to the development of its public health system. The "green gold" of henequen transformed Yucatán into one of Mexico's wealthiest states. Close-knit political elite (the *casta divina*) monopolized this economic dynamo and defended henequen production from would-be critics—either domestic or foreign. Yucatec officials established public health programs as a strategy for the modernization of the region, using wealth from the production of henequen to create one of Mexico's most extensive public health systems, notably under the auspices of the social assistance program of the *Henequeneros de Yucatán* (1938–1955). The collapse of fiber prices after the Second World War led to the bankruptcy of the *Henequeneros de Yucatán* and the incorporation of its public health program into the federal medical network.

The scholarly literature in medical anthropology and the history of medicine and science has expanded rapidly over the past generation.[4] The transformation has been so fundamental that Anne-Emanuelle Birn argues "that studies of health and society are poised to go from a subspecialty to a pillar of Latin American research and teaching—potentially serving as a fulcrum of social, political, and cultural history."[5]

Scholars of the history of medicine have generated a distinct lexicon and multiple theoretical orientations, much of which are reflected in this work. The anthropologist Irwin Press, who studied Piste, a small town in Yucatán, and Bogotá, Colombia, explored the concept of a "medical system" that sought to avoid the inherent hierarchical biases evident in the work of Redfield and others who utilize a modernizationist theoretical approach. For

Press, a medical system is "a patterned, interrelated body of values and deliberate practices, governed by a single paradigm of meaning, identification, prevention, and treatment of sickness."[6] The "single paradigm" is critical to Press's concept of a medical system. Humoralism, for example, envisions the body to be composed of four humors that must be kept in balance for a state of good health. An illness produced by too much "heat" requires a "cold" treatment, usually a particular food or set of herbs. A "disease narrative" of symptoms, diagnosis, treatment and prognosis would explain all illnesses using this paradigm of meaning, and give fundamental insight into the medical system. Medical systems can be simple or complex, depending largely upon the size of the infrastructure that supports it. The "biomedical" system that dominates most of the Atlantic World is quite complex, with a huge range of institutional, social, political, and economic facets. "Medical pluralism" implies the presence of several distinct approaches to healing in a particular society; for example, in China, illnesses are treated through Chinese traditional medicine, biomedicine, and other paradigms. This medical system conceptualization enables the study of medical ideologies, or disease narratives, through comparative research lenses.

The medical system constructed in Yucatán after the 1870s relied upon a biomedical approach to healing. Biomedicine envisions the body to be a biomechanical system; illnesses can be caused by agents such as germs or viruses, or perhaps functional deficiencies of the body. The biomedical body is part of the natural world as understood by Enlightenment scholars, governed by natural laws that can be determined by scientific investigations. Illnesses are usually treated by specialists trained in knowledge generated by the experiential method. William Harvey's understanding of the heart (1628) as a "pump" illustrates the mechanical vision of the body; just as his rejection of "inherited" knowledge in favor of first-hand investigation and extensive use of vivisection reveals the scientific method. Louis Pasteur's and Robert Koch's development of germ theory in the 1870s and 1880s enabled the identification of the origins of many diseases, as well as the means to develop vaccines that could kill or inhibit germs. Germ theory led to the laboratory becoming a primary source of knowledge generation. In late-nineteenth-century Yucatán, public health organizations reproduced the development of rabies vaccine, and helped in the pursuit of the "germ" of yellow fever, all facets of a biomedical system.

The development of biomedicine created new patterns of knowledge and new sources of power. Michel Foucault's works on the clinic and the panopticon enabled him to develop the concept of "biopower."[7] The nineteenth-century French clinic for the destitute became a site where physicians learned about illnesses from the study of poor bodies—often through morbid anatomy—and applied their knowledge to treat more well-to-do citizens.

This leads to two of Foucault's important contributions—the gaze and his sense of the social contract. Social contract suggests the power relationship between the elite and the poor, wherein poor bodies can be treated and utilized as sources of healing that can then be used by the elite patrons of clinical knowledge. By gaze, Foucault implies the ability of the physician with anatomoclinical knowledge to "see" a disease inside or outside the body; this gaze objectifies the ill individual into a "diseased object" knowable by the physician.[8]

Another power of the gaze is visible in the Jeremy Bentham's vision of the panopticon. The hub and spoke layout of the panopticon—in which prisoners could not see their supervisors, but guards could see all prisoners at any time—engendered a sense in the minds of prisoners that they might be watched at any time, an internalization of constant surveillance that changed their behavior. Similarly, biopower engendered concepts of normalcy—oftentimes expressed in terms of the body or gender conduct that structured social behavior. The importance of statistics and standard deviations to define normalcy pervades the pioneering work of Francis Galton and became integral to the eugenic movement and to biomedical testing. Having defined the norm, biopower can assign deviancy—departures from the "norm." The IQ test, for example, was developed in the early twentieth-century United States to assess persons with mental illnesses; deviancy became integral to the eugenic analysis of race. Our blood tests rely upon normative values to indicate "good" or "high" levels of broad range of characteristics, such as our cholesterol levels. We almost unconsciously understand test results as reflecting our normalcy or risk factors, a clear outcome of how biopower creates our sense of good or poor health. Biopower causes the internalization of knowledge, and alters behavior into what might be understood to be normal.

Several historiographic trends dominated the history of medicine prior to the 1980s. A heroic genre often produced by physicians tended to glorify the "firsts" and the "famous," detailing the inevitable march of medical progress, such as depicted in the works of Mexico's Miguel Bustamante.[9] A Marxist approach either critiqued internal structures of power or examined patterns of international economic relationships using the language of core-periphery dependency. Outside Marxist scholarship, medical and political centers dominated the history of public health in Latin America, with studies historically focused upon the institutional activities of central governments, national health initiatives, or upon the role of powerful international organizations such as the Rockefeller Foundation. This pattern of scholarship parallels the power relationship imbedded in the contemporary system of international public health, which links organizations such as the World Health Organization to national governments, which in turn dominate national public health systems. This approach was facilitated by the relative abundance of documents produced by national and international bureaucracies, and the tendency to use historical analyses to demonstrate medical "progress."

While the heroic genre has been marginalized, the attention to center/periphery relationships has survived, albeit with substantive modifications. Adrián López-Denis suggests that centers in the Atlantic medical community might better be seen as a series of changing nodes of knowledge, technologies, and authorities, and that peripheries be envisioned in shifting relationships to centers.[10] In a collection of essays honoring the path-setting scholarship of Nancy Stepan, Anne-Emanuelle Birn and Raúl Necochea López observe that

> Newer studies of the local-global nexus in Latin America recognize international health to be a dynamic arena in which local actors (unions, healers, residents, or political authorities), national politicians, researchers and policy specialists, transnational professionals, and international agencies interact and mold one another.[11]

The rigidity of the dependency paradigm has been replaced by nuance, complexity, reciprocity, and attention to place and time—though all within the power structures of the Atlantic world.

Medicine on the Periphery envisages an Atlantic medical community with shifting centers, peripheries, and nodes of power/authority. The perspective from Yucatán is of a "flatter" nineteenth-century Atlantic medical community, with technologies and knowledge more easily adopted and utilized by medical practitioners throughout the region. The relative autonomy of Yucatán's early public health system fits within this conception. So too do the *Escola Tropicalista Bahiana* and the *Instituto Oswaldo Cruz*,[12] both of which produced medical knowledge principally intended for Brazil, with fewer intellectual debts to the scientific core. Steven Palmer argues that a Cuban bacteriological institute founded in 1885 played a similar role.[13]

Yucatán can be seen as an early center that lost autonomy over the course of the twentieth century. Other countries or regions that had served as medical nodes—such as Cuba—experienced relational changes from centers to peripheries, as powerful actors such as the United States altered the environments in which local or national policies might prevail.[14] The development of the Mexican state and the transformation of the biomedical industry accounts for Yucatán's shift toward peripheral status. The expansion of national health bureaucracies such as the Mexican Social Security Institute (*Instituto Mexicano de Seguro Social*, IMSS, 1943), coupled with the collapse of the henequen industry, weakened Yucatán's capacity to assert its own priorities. By the mid-twentieth century, knowledge and biomedical technologies had become increasingly capitalized, complex, and less easy to replicate. In Yucatán, as will be seen, this process is visible in the pages of medical journals, which in the early 1900s offered recipes that would enable physicians to produce their own drugs, but became the purview of pharmaceutical companies such as Eli Lilly and Wellcome by the 1940s. In contexts such as Yucatán, new nodes of power created peripheries in consuming regions increasingly dependent upon knowledge and technologies produced in the productive core of the North Atlantic.

The new historiography has reconfigured the relationship between the Rockefeller Foundation and Latin American nations. Scholars in Marcos Cueto's 1994 *Missionaries of Science* moved away from the "top-down" understanding penned by officials working with the Foundation, to focus upon local and national actors,[15] inspiring others to study this vital international agency and its role within Latin American public health systems. Notable works are Palmer's *Launching Global Health: The Caribbean Odyssey of the Rockefeller Foundation* and Birn's *Marriage of Convenience: Rockefeller International Health and Revolutionary Mexico*. Palmer details Rockefeller's efforts to transport its anti-hookworm campaign from the US South into the circum-Caribbean, a process marked by tremendous levels of cooperation (and tensions) between national governments and the potent US Foundation.[16] *Marriage of Convenience* painstakingly traces the efforts by the Foundation to gain access to nationalist Mexico, and the institutional dance as both partners sought the primacy of their priorities. The cooperative relationship led to campaigns against yellow fever, hookworm, and malaria,[17] and cooperative health units in Vera cruz.[18] (These units would model the health programs installed in nationalized *ejidos* under the Cárdenas administration.) As Palmer suggests, the roles of local officials, such as the Yucatec *Junta Superior de Sanidad*, are often overshadowed by the mammoth Rockefeller Foundation, as will be seen in the campaign against yellow fever in Yucatán.

Students of Yucatec medical history owe a tremendous debt to Eduardo L. Menéndez. His seminal *Poder, estratificación y salud* (1981) is a model of Marxist critical anthropology. Menéndez offers a detailed analysis of illnesses in the 1970s, an overview of institutions of healing in the twentieth century, and a powerful rejection of the "traditional/modern" paradigm favored by scholars inspired by the community studies approach of Redfield. For Menéndez, the socio political system spawned by the production of henequen is central to the medical reality of Yucatec residents produced by henequen and capitalism.[19]

Medicine on the Periphery de-centers the study of public health, even as relations among peripheries and centers remain critical points of analysis. The stimuli to create a Yucatec public health network originated in Yucatán, not with the revolutionary Mexican state, the leading cities of the Atlantic powers, or the boardrooms of powerful international agencies. Yucatec officials viewed their efforts to develop a public health system as part of the sanitation movement that was transforming the Atlantic medical community. The regional elite who managed public health programs in Yucatán were well aware of international tendencies, but applied them in ways that reflected their own values. They had a limited commitment to a broad program of public health, preferring to focus upon urban as opposed to rural conditions, and offering services to white, as opposed to Maya residents of the state. The multi faceted Atlantic medical community was more central to the region's public health system than that of the Mexican government. Yucatán was not subject to the exploitive forces of tropical, imperial medicine, nor manipulated by agencies such as the International Health Board (IHB) of the Rockefeller Foundation. External forces—including the Mexican government—shaped Yucatec public health, but not to the point of domination until after the 1950s.

This history of public health in Yucatán stresses locality; the perspectives and activities of Yucatec officials occupy center stage. The federal government occupied a decidedly secondary position through the 1930s, when the revolutionary state impacted Yucatec structures in dramatic—though not yet domineering—fashion. However, by the 1950s, when the henequen bonanza came to a definitive end, and when the nature of the Atlantic medical community had changed, the primacy of Yucatec public health leadership came to an end, becoming more peripheral to both the Mexican state and external sources of biomedical knowledge. The "biomedicalization" of Yucatán implies a truly transformative process. A new medical system, replete with physicians with a distinct body of knowledge and ways of healing, and a complex institutional infrastructure developed after the 1870s.

Institutions, diseases, medical practitioners, and the activities of public health agencies give organizational structure to *Medicine on the Periphery*. The initial chapter "sets the stage," offering an overview of Yucatec history from the Spanish conquest, through the radical changes engendered by the Caste War and the emergence of the henequen economy, the emergence of Mérida as the state's leading urban center, and changing patterns of health care. Subsequent chapters develop various dimensions of the public health project.

Medical institutions are examined in the second chapter. Mérida's School of Medicine, founded in 1833, produced hundreds of physicians who practiced in the region, serving as a principle source of medical knowledge for the region. A general hospital that combined two colonial institutions emerged in mid-century, eventually becoming the Hospital O'Horán (1906), an imposing complex that highlighted the modernization of Yucatec medical facilities. Physicians founded a series of professional organizations to represent themselves as superior to other medical practitioners, organizations that served as valuable conduits to medical communities in Buenos Aires, Mexico

City, Havana, Paris, London, and elsewhere. The state's *Junta Superior de Sanidad* began with an extensive set of responsibilities largely limited to the capital and the key port of Progreso. In time, the body would extend its service throughout the state through auxiliary health boards and would guide the social assistance program of the *Henequeneros de Yucatán*. The second chapter concludes with an analysis of the changing activities of the *Junta Superior de Sanidad*, suggesting priorities articulated by Yucatec officials and the growing influence of the Mexican state.

A biomedical healing community developed over the course of the nineteenth century, coming to dominate statewide healing practices by the end of the twentieth century. This is the focus of chapter 3. It opens with a consideration of the colonial world of healers, and then draws upon anthropological studies to survey Yucatán's range of healers in the first half of the twentieth century. Most of the chapter develops an analysis of five medical "generations"—Founding, Professionalizing, Institutionalizing, Revolutionary, and Specialist. Tracing the knowledge, public health concerns, and priorities of these generations demonstrates the active role of physicians in the creation of the new medical system of Yucatán. Critical to that process was the move to gain exclusive authority to practice medicine, the creation of public health institutions as vehicles of corporate power, and the development of solidarities with national and international medical communities.

The response to diseases changed dramatically with new medical knowledge and the development of public health programs in the nineteenth century. The great colonial killers of indigenous peoples—smallpox, influenza, and various fevers—could not be controlled save by sporadic and ineffective quarantines, and perhaps appeals to divine intervention. These measures were equally ineffective against new diseases with less racial discrimination—yellow fever after 1648 and cholera after the 1830s. The development of a small pox vaccination program in the early 1800s and international agreements to coordinate reactions to cholera suggested the potential of biomedical practitioners to limit the ravages of disease. Chapter 4 examines these topics, and considers in detail the campaigns by the *Junta Superior de Sanidad* and other agencies against a broad range of diseases, including small pox, yellow fever, and tuberculosis. In part due to these interventions, the state experienced an "epidemiological transition" that transformed the region's disease landscape, leading to the decline of deaths due to contagious diseases and reduction in infant mortality, and the subsequent increase of more chronic illnesses as the principal causes of death.

Chapter 5 treats the relationship between state and federal public health programs. It introduces the nineteenth-century federal effort to consolidate colonial structures and, under the leadership of Eduardo Liceaga (1829–1920), to modernize the organization and scope of federal agencies. Far more dramatic changes took place in the wake of the Revolution, when the "right" to health was instilled within the Constitution of 1917. In the 1920s, the DSP attempted—with little early success—to assert its authority over state public health agencies, a move that met much resistance in Yucatán. The vast expansion of *ejidos* under Cárdenas in the 1930s included the creation of public health agencies as means of modernizing rural citizens. Yucatec henequen elite unsuccessfully attempted to block the nationalization of their properties, but created the *Henequeneros de Yucatán*, which kept marketing of the fiber under control. The social assistance program of the *Henequeneros* allowed for a dramatic expansion of health care facilities in the henequen zone, a program that eventually served one in three Yucatec residences. Federal officials did institute public health offices in newly created *ejidos* in the corn zone, as well as the UN *Bienestar Rural* initiative. By the 1950s, Yucatán had Mexico's most extensive system of rural health care, but also the most precarious, in that it relied upon the price of fiber in the commodity market. The collapse of those prices led to the demise of the *Henequeneros de Yucatán* in 1955 and the nationalization of its health care system.

Biomedicalization built upon an expanding infrastructure, a potent corps of practitioners, increased efficacy, and the process of state formation to dominate Yucatec medical practices by the 1950s. Chapter 6 examines three dimensions of biomedicalization. The first treats the Maya-dominated "interior" of the state, and its transition from "traditional" medicine, to medical pluralism, and finally to biomedical domination. The second section addresses the impact of biomedicine upon the disease profile of the state and the epidemiologic transition that occurred over the course of the twentieth century. Yucatec public health within the context of the Atlantic medical community reveals an apparent paradox: the gradual transformation of Yucatán from a relatively autonomous center of public health activity to a medical periphery vis-à-vis Mexican and North Atlantic medical communities. The process of peripheralization of Yucatán is common to much of the world, suggesting the capacity of biopower to shape the lives of most residents of the planet.

NOTES

1. Nelson A. Reed, *The Caste War of Yucatán,* revised ed. (Stanford: Stanford University Press, 2001).

2. Robert Redfield, *The Folk Culture of Yucatan* (Chicago: University of Chicago Press, 1941). The word "tradition" is laden with multiple meanings that are generally juxtaposed with "modernity," itself complicated by various interpretations. For Redfield, the two occupy distinct ends of a historical spectrum that leads from a primitive past to a modern present. Social tensions accompany the movement along

this historical path. This concept will be treated (and criticized) in the context in chapter 6.

3. David Sowell, *The Tale of Healer Miguel Perdomo Neira: Medicine, Ideologies, and Power in the Nineteenth-Century Andes* (Wilmington, DE: Scholarly Resources, 2001).

4. Historiographic essays include Ann Zulawski, "New Trends in Studies of Science and Medicine in Latin America," *Latin American Research Review* 34:3 (1999), 241-51; Anne-Emanuelle Birn, "Healers, Healing, and Child Well-Being: Ideologies, Institutions, and Health in Latin America and the Caribbean," *Latin American Research Review* 40:2 (June 2005), 176-92; Diego Armus, "Disease in the Historiography of Modern Latin America," in *From Malaria to Aids: Disease in the History of Modern Latin America*, ed. by Diego Armus (Durham: Duke University Press, 2003), 1-24; Amy Whitfield and Howard Waitzkin, "The Vicissitudes of Public Health Policy in the Americas," *Latin American Research Review* 44:2 (2009), 216–24; Julia Rodríguez and Ann Zulawski, "Science and Medicine in Latin America," *Hispanic American Historical Review* (Special Edition: "Science and Medicine in Latin America," essays in Honor of Nancy Leys Stepan) 91:3 (August 2011), 387–408; and Steven Palmer and Claudia Agostoni, "Introduction: Landscapes of Latin American Health, 1870–1970," *Canadian Journal of Latin American and Caribbean Studies* 35:69 (2010), 5–18.

5. Birn, "Healers, Healing, and Child Well-Being," 192.

6. Irwin Press, "Problems in the Definition and Classification of Medical Systems," *Social Science and Medicine* 1:14B (1980), 47.

7. Michel Foucault, *The History of Sexuality: The Will to Knowledge*, trans. by Robert Hurley (New York, Vintage Books, 1990), 140.

8. Foucault, *The Birth of the Clinic: An Archeology of Medical Perception*, trans. by A. M. Sheridan Smith (New York: Vintage/Random House, 1994).

9. Miguel E. Bustamante, *Cinco personajes de la salud en México* (México DF: Grupo Editorial Angel Porrúa, 1986).

10. Adrián López-Denis, "Comments on the Panel "Between Foreign Approaches and Domestic Priorities: The Forging of International Health in Twentieth Century Latin America" (paper presented at XXIX International Congress of the Latin American Studies Association, Toronto Canada, October 6–9, 2010).

11. Birn and Raúl Neocochea López, "Footprints in the Future: Looking Forward to the History of Health and Medicine in Latin America in the Twenty-First Century," *Hispanic American Historical Review* 91:3 (August 2011), 518.

12. Julyan G. Peard, *Race, Place, and Medicine: The Idea of the Tropics in Nineteenth Century Brazilian Medicine* (Durham, NC: Duke University Press, 1999). On Oswaldo Cruz, see Nancy Stepan, *Beginnings of Brazilian Science: Oswaldo Cruz, Medical Research and Policy, 1890–1920* (New York: Science History Publications, 1981) and Jaime L. Benchimol, ed., *Manguihos, do sonho à vida: A ciência na Belle Époque* (Rio de Janeiro: Casa de Oswaldo Cruz, 1990).

13. Steven Palmer "Beginnings of Cuban Bacteriology: Juan Santos Fernández, Medical Research, and the Search for Scientific Sovereignty, 1880–1920," *Hispanic American Historical Review* 91:3 (August 2011), 445–68.

14. Mariola Espinosa, *Epidemic Invasions: Yellow Fever and the Limits of Cuban Independence, 1878-1930* (Chicago: The University of Chicago Press, 2009); Palmer, "Beginnings of Cuban Bacteriology," 445–468.

15. Marcos Cueto, ed., *Missionaries of Science: The Rockefeller Foundation and Latin America* (Bloomington: Indiana University Press, 1994).

16. Steven Palmer, *Launching Global Health: The Caribbean Odyssey of the Rockefeller Foundation* (Ann Arbor: University of Michigan Press, 2010).

17. Cueto, *Cold War, Deadly Fevers: Malaria Eradication in Mexico, 1955-75* (Baltimore: The Johns Hopkins University Press, 2007).

18. Birn, *Marriage of Convenience: Rockefeller International Health and Revolutionary Mexico* (Rochester: University of Rochester Press, 2006).

19. Eduardo L. Menéndez, *Poder, estratificación y salud: Análisis de las condiciones sociales y económicas de la enfermedad en Yucatán* (Mexico City DF: Ediciones de las Casa Chata, 1981).

Acknowledgments

Students, colleagues, archivists, and librarians facilitated the research for this work and greatly improved its quality. The staffs of the Archivo General del Yucatan, the Biblioteca Yucatense, and the Yucatán room in the library of the Universidad Autónoma de Yucatán were open and giving to a new student of Yucatán. In Mexico City, archivists at the Archivo Histórico de la Escuela de Medicina, Archivo Histórico de la Secretaría de Salubridad y Asistencia, and Archivo General Nacional proved especially helpful. Raymundo Telix Alvárez García, Rocio Romero Hernández provided invaluable assistance at the AGN. The staff at the College of Physicians of Philadelphia, Historical Medical Library, Philadelphia, Pennsylvania, were very welcoming. Research assistants at the National Library of Medicine, and Mary Ann Quinn at the Rockefeller Archive Center in Sleepy Hollow, New York guided me through their excellent collections.

The University Center for International Studies, University of Pittsburgh, supported my Summer Research Fellowship in Latin American Studies. Rosalind Santavicca and Luis Bravo facilitated my time in Pittsburgh. John Erlin, Director of History of Medicine Collection, Falk Library of the Health Sciences at the University of Pittsburgh has been an ongoing aid to this project.

Juniata College has supported this research through the William J. and Francis Nyce Fund and the Dave Goodman Summer Research Fund. Provost Jim Lakso provided special assistance. Student Lauren Chambers was wonderfully supportive as we shared the Goodman award. Amy Hunt provided invaluable assistance making sure that my notes and bibliography matched. Emily Tone assisted with the construction of the index. My colleagues Dave Hsiung and Belle Tuten have offered many kind comments.

I gratefully acknowledge Routledge Press for permission to use materials from my article "Race and the Authorization of Biomedicine in Yucatán,

Mexico," in *Health and Medicine in the Circum-Caribbean, 1800–1968*, ed. by Juanita De Barros, Steven Palmer, and David Wright (New York: Routledge Press, 2009). Additionally, select materials in chapters 2, 5, and 6 were originally published in "Multiple Colonizations: State Formation, Public Health and the Yucatec Maya, 1891–1960," by David Sowell, in *Crossing Colonial Historiographies: Histories of Colonial and Indigenous Medicines in Transnational Perspective*, eds. Anne Digby, Waltraud Ernst, and Projit B. Muchkarji (Cambridge UK: Cambridge Scholars Inc., 2010), 77–97.

Over the years, a variety of colleagues have read portions of the manuscript or shared comments on panels. I would single out the assistance of Anne-Emanuel Birn, Marcos Cueto, Adrián López-Denis, Julia Rodriguez, Allen Wells, and members of the PA Yucatán roundtable organized by Matthew Restall.

My family has lived with this project for some time—at times peacefully, and at times with considerable consternation. Emily has read many sections, and with her insightful eye caught many errors and points that needed clarification. Chris has suffered through many trips to archives, conferences, and talks that took me away from our joyful time together. It is a pleasure to dedicate this work to the life that she envisioned for us.

Chapter 1

Public Health and the Making of Modern Yucatán

By late 1939, tuberculosis had so sickened Secundina Reye that she could no longer take care of herself. Public health officials associated with the collectively owned henequen *ejido* of Xcanatún notified their superiors in Mérida of her condition. Dr. Carlos Mendoza, head of the Department of Health and Beneficience (*Departamento de Beneficencia y Sanidad*), visited Reye's home and confirmed the severity of the illness. Since her *na*—the traditional Mayan thatched hut—was near the center of the *ejido* and close to other houses, Mendoza recommended that Reye be placed in isolation at the *Hospital O'Horán* in Mérida and that her house be burned, insofar as it could not be disinfected.[1] We do not know Reye's fate, but do know that tuberculosis caused the death of many Yucatec residents in both rural and urban settings.

Mendoza and Reye occupied different points in what might have been Mexico's most extensive public health system in the 1930s. Yucatán's initial sanitarian effort by the *Junta Superior de Sanidad* focused upon the capital city of Mérida and included the 1906 construction of the Hospital O'Horán, where Reye was treated. In time, public health officials extended their efforts to rural dwellers in keeping with the revolutionary objectives of the Constitution of 1917. Yucatec officials managed the social assistance program of the *Henequeneros de Yucatán* that served scores of rural communities such as Xcanatún through permanently staffed clinics; even more residents in the henequen zone had periodic access to nurses and physicians. Toward the end of the 1950s, Yucatán housed 29 percent of the country's regional health centers, 59 percent of its Unified Sanitary Units, and 74 percent of its First Aid Posts. Most rural Yucatec residents had access to a public health facility,[2] and traditional medicine was in rapid retreat before the power of biomedicine.

This case speaks to a remarkable sequence of events made possible by the radical transformation of Yucatán after the 1870s. The fiber of the henequen plant underpinned that transformation, becoming the source of remarkable wealth that sparked a Yucatec "golden age." Henequen, a member of the agave family, grows fibrous leaves capable of producing a sturdy twine. Demand from the United States and Canadian wheat industry spurred the nineteenth-century construction of scores of henequen estates in northwest Yucatán and transformation of the state. Yucatec elite pursued an aggressive modernization project, to demonstrate not only that they were part of the Mexican mainstream, but also that they could act independent of political forces of central Mexico.[3]

Henequen blessed only a small number of Yucatec residents however. Thousands labored in conditions of near-slavery, many of them *ejido* residents such as Reye. The behavior of the henequen elite angered many, especially after the Mexican Revolution challenged the social, economic, and political power that privileged large landowners. Revolutionary officials were unable to curb the power of the henequen elite until the 1930s, when the federal government seized the estates and created hundreds of henequen *ejidos*—lands held in collective ownership by laborers. President Lázaro Cárdenas's regime (1934–1940) insisted that all *ejido* residents have access to health care, leading to the creation of the "Social Assistance" program of the *Henequeneros de Yucatán* by the state government. Contrary to the objectives of the revolutionary government, former landowners of the henequen plantations dominated the *Henequeneros*, continuing to market the fiber and assert considerable control over their recently expropriated properties. Still, the social assistance program of the *Henequeneros* delivered health care to *ejido* residents and salaried henequen workers.

The construction of a public health system was central to the creation of modern Yucatán. This introduction provides an overview of the Yucatec context, highlighting the social and political environments in which public health efforts developed. It considers three broad periods: the colonial era, the "second conquest" from the 1780s through the Caste War, and the emergence of "modern" Yucatán after the 1860s. The "white city" of Mérida, site of many public health initiatives, merits special attention. This overview thus sets the stage for the analysis of the biomedical system explored in later chapters.

THE COLONIAL WORLD

Yucatán occupied a peripheral position within the Viceroyalty of New Spain. Lacking valuable resources and dense native populations, settlers, missionaries, and natives settled into an uneasy relationship that persisted through most of the colonial era. Old World diseases caused tremendous losses among native peoples, though their communities retained sufficient autonomy to maintain many pre-Columbian cultural traits. Spanish characteristics dominated urban places, external relations, racialized social structures, and public religious practices. Hispanic medical practices shaped indigenous responses to disease, especially in religious terms, but had less direct impact on the daily lives of the indigene, demonstrating the superficiality of Spanish influence upon the social and cultural norms of the native population. This colonial medical heritage persisted well into the twentieth century in areas whites would call the "interior," the last zones to become part of the biomedical community.

Colonial Yucatán encompassed the present-day Mexican states of Campeche, Quintana Roo, and Yucatán. Within this vast expanse were striking social, economic, and geographic variations. Yucatán's demography and geography dictated at least three regions: the thin-soiled northwest, dominated by Mérida and Izamal; the more fertile lands to the south and east, dominated by Valladolid, Tekax, and the port of Campeche; and, further to the south, a forested zone leading to the jungles of Petén. Whites, mestizos, and a small but important number of Africans were concentrated in Campeche, the capital of Mérida, and Valladolid.[4] Elsewhere, small Maya hamlets and villages were the norm.

In all but the forested south, *milpas* dominated agricultural production. The *milpa* is a small plot of land cleared in the scrub land, its wood burned as fertilizer, and planted for two or three years. Though communities held the land in common, *milpas* were grown by families, and might be several kilometers from the village. As the *milpa* lost fertility, a new plot would be burned, and the old one allowed lay to fallow for ten to fifteen years. Spaniards introduced cattle ranching, but *milpa* agriculture dominated until well into the nineteenth century. After the 1860s, large-scale henequen estates would dominate the northeast (the henequen zone) and *milpa* production of corn would continue to dominate the more fertile eastern and southern areas (the corn zone).

Spaniard and Maya viewed themselves and each other differently. For the Spaniards, the Maya were *indios*, a colonial label that reflected the racialized Hispanic worldview. The only *indio* subset for the Spaniards was some 200 "Indian nobles." Spaniards saw differences among themselves, especially whether one had been born in Spain, central Mexico, or in Yucatán. Spaniards were still one race, unified by their Christian civilization, albeit with occasionally competing interests, especially vis-à-vis control of indigenous labor. By contrast, indigenous identity was rooted in the *cah* (community), and not to a common ethnicity. *Cah* leaders (*batab*) might well be descendants of preconquest lineages, though this tended to be less common over time. Maya tended to refer to themselves as *masewales*, a term that implied commoners, or poor people. Not until the Caste War of the nineteenth century would a broader identity develop among some Maya. To the Maya, all Spaniards were *dzules* (foreigners or whites), a term that would persist through the twentieth century. Mestizos were closely associated with the Spanish world, often linking the Spanish and Maya worlds. A small number of *mulatos* and *pardos* lived in the Campeche region. Mestizos, *mulatos*, and *pardos* might be referred to as "half white" (*k'as dzul*) by the Maya.[5]

Grant Jones reminds students of Yucatec history that the northern lowlands dominated by Mérida were "the land of foreigners" to many Maya. The *Books of Chilam Balam* spoke to the inevitability of conquest, disasters, and enslavement in this region. Only in this zone did the Spaniards establish an effective colonial system. In the jungles of southern Yucatán, conquest and colonization occurred quite differently. Not until the late seventeenth century were the autonomous southern zones conquered, and even then, colonization developed quite differently than in northern Yucatán. As a result, for well over 100 years after Mérida had come to dominate the north, a frontier zone signaled the boundary of effective Spanish colonial authority and autonomous Maya communities. The northern zone constituted a Spanish frontier to many Maya; the southern zone a frontier to the Spanish.[6]

The Catholic Church provided much of the cohesion for the peninsula. Colonizers were concentrated in the cities, where small secular churches served Spanish needs; Franciscan missionaries undertook evangelical work throughout the peninsula. From their "headquarters" in Izamal, some eighty parishes divided the region by the end of the colonial period. Parish priests worked closely with community leaders; clerical fees accompanied baptisms, marriages, and deaths. These fees enabled many *curas* to develop extensive land holdings, as well to sustain convents and clerical offices in Mérida, Izamal, Mani, and elsewhere. Franciscans helped to found *cofradias* among the various Maya communities, each of which invariably hosted a church, whether a *cura* sat in residence or not.

Spanish conquerors imposed a system of tribute labor that supported a small-scale hacienda system. Haciendas produced cattle, corn, and other foodstuffs, mostly for local markets. Spaniards gradually took over the valuable salt flats of the northern coast, using salt for both internal and export sales. Although Campeche served as the point of export for hides and salt, the region produced little more than it could consume, and little that was in demand elsewhere. "Yucatán's poverty," in the words of Inga Clendinnen, "protected it from sustained attention from the crown"[7] and, over time, sustained a regional identity distinct from that of central Mexico.

The Spanish *encomienda* system dictated that Maya communities provide periodic laborers for their haciendas, a system that did not fundamentally alter community life. *Vaqueros* worked for the cattle estates, but many natives in northwest Yucatán produced corn on hacienda land in exchange for periodic labor. For most of the colonial period, the maintenance of native communities meant that most Maya remained "*indios del pueblo.*" Only in the late colonial period, with the intensification of the hacienda system, did they become "*peones de hacienda,*" the eventual laborers for the henequen estates.[8]

A "*pacto colonial*" governed relationships between Maya and Spaniards. The allocation of Maya peoples as *encomienda* laborers satisfied a principle objective of the colonizers. In exchange, Maya were able to preserve "important spaces of autonomous life, spaces that were indispensable for the maintenance of their cultural dynamic and the preservation and recreation of their own social organization, which permitted [the Maya] to conserve a distinct identity over the long term."[9] The *pacto colonial* enabled Maya *batab* to serve as intermediaries between indigenous communities and the Spaniards.[10] It permitted the *cah* to persist as both a primary source of identity and a geopolitical entity throughout the colonial period.[11]

COLONIAL HEALTH INSTITUTIONS

Conquest altered the demography of Yucatán. Perhaps 800,000 people occupied the peninsula at contact. European diseases played a primary role in reducing that number to about 185,000 tribute-paying Maya by 1605, at the same time that just over 7,000 Spaniards, mestizos, and others lived in the peninsula. Indigenous numbers continued to decline until the 1750s, after which they increased rapidly until the Caste War of the 1840s. The eighteenth century saw a dramatic increase in the non-Maya population, to an estimate of over 100,000 by the 1790s, some 29 percent of the total population of 357,000. In 1794, the region around Mérida totaled almost 28,000 people, 47 percent of whom were non-Indians; only 25 percent of the town dwellers were Indians.[12]

The *protomedicato* and the Church dominated official Hispanic medical institutions throughout the Indies. The *protomedicato*, a Royal Board of Health, regulated and licensed physicians, responded to epidemic diseases, and inspected apothecary shops, all under the authorization of the crown, a hierarchy that kept health care under executive authority. However, the limited extension of direct crown influence in many areas of the Indies led urban municipal councils (*cabildos*) to fulfill the functions of the *protomedicato*. Hospitals and church-led beneficence agencies constituted another important range of medical institutions in New Spain. For most residents, church affiliates constituted the most likely direct contact with institutionalized medicine.

In Yucatán, these institutional structures barely functioned. The yellow fever outbreak in 1648 illustrates their weaknesses. The disease first struck Campeche in June, spread to Mérida in August, Valladolid in September, and eventually reached most villages of the region. Residents complained of fevers and chills, aches in various areas of their bodies, fatigue, and nausea. For many, vomiting blood (the fabled black vomit), jaundiced skin, and a painful death followed initial symptoms. Spaniards were especially fearful of the disease, as most previous epidemics had afflicted primarily the native populations. This epidemic spared no one. The governor died from the disease, along with large numbers of resident Franciscans and Jesuits. By the time it subsided in 1650, perhaps half of the population had died.[13]

Explanations for the disease varied. Many indigenous residents no doubt figured it to be one in a long line of illnesses that had struck the region since the arrival of the Spaniards, an interpretation in line with pre-Columbian cosmological understandings. Franciscan priest and scholar Diego López de Cogolludo thought that God was punishing residents for their evil ways. The governor likely thought along similar lines, for he ordered the Virgin of Izamal brought to the capital to cure its residents, a desperate move that failed to alleviate the outbreak. Hispanic physicians were baffled, having no knowledge of this type of disease.[14] Indeed, aside from prayers and the imposition of quarantines, physicians of the day had few measures that might lessened the suffering of the ill. Unfortunately, once established, yellow fever ravaged the peninsula with alarming frequency.

The appearance of yellow fever in 1648 suggests two Yucatec healing traditions: one centered among colonized indigene and the other that of the conquerors. Maya accounts reflected upon the disease as one of many calamities that had accompanied conquest, which were treated by a corps of healers with localized power. Spaniards responded to the disease with a blend of humoral-based practices, religious beliefs, and a sparse institutional apparatus, always associated with the Church. (The Church established a series of small hospitals after 1547 that offered more spiritual than medical care.)[15] For either the colonizer or colonized, it would be quite difficult to distinguish between religious and lay beliefs about disease and healing, characteristics that enabled a slow melding of healing beliefs. Public policy resided firmly in Hispanic hands and focused primarily upon isolation and quarantine of diseased persons. The capacity to control diseases or reduce their severity was limited.

The *pacto colonial* meant that many preconquest medical patterns persisted in a colonized space. Maya healers operated within boundaries established by the Catholic Church, so that *ah-men* (healers) could not perform public rituals that priests might find idolatrous. Healing ideologies nevertheless drew deeply upon earlier traditions, especially in the use of medicinal plants. In the mid-sixteenth century, Franciscan Diego de Landa noted the use of "great quantities of medicinal plants," but did not record their properties or discuss the healers who prescribed them. Numerous Maya accounts from the colonial period discuss plants and healers, notably in the various *Books of Chilam Balam* (especially those from Ixil). The mid-eighteenth-century *Yerbas y hechicerías del Yucatán* appears to have recorded plants and healers in the Valladolid region. This pattern of herbal use and preconquest medical influences lasted until well into the twentieth century.[16] (Discussed in chapter 3.)

THE SECOND CONQUEST

The efforts by Bourbon monarchs after 1763 to develop commodity markets and increase revenues in the Indies triggered a "second conquest" of Yucatán. The Bourbon Reforms ended the period of indirect crown rule, altering norms for Spaniard and Maya alike. The reforms stimulated an economic revival, involving sugar in some regions and cattle ranching in others. The reforms sparked dramatic changes in the social, economic, and political landscapes of Yucatán in the seventy years after the 1780s.[17]

Actions of the Bourbon reformers spelled the end of the *pacto colonial*.[18] In seeking to make their empire more profitable, administratively responsive, and more defensible, the Bourbon administrators redrew the political boundaries of Yucatán into fifteen *partidos* in 1786, each centered on a town or city. Most of these *partidos* persisted well into the twentieth century. Some fell into the jurisdiction of Campeche, which became an independent state in 1858. Others were part of Quintana Roo, which too became a separate state in the twentieth century. (Twentieth-century public health officials used these *partidos* as their basic unit of reference.)

The governor of Yucatán presided over a new corps of officials. Subdelegates each had jurisdiction over a *partido* and reported directly to the governor. *Subdelgados* labored with Spanish judges (*jueces españoles*), especially in the collection of taxes. Direct rule replaced the indirect rule of the *pacto colonial*, leading to frequent interventions by Spaniards in the Maya communities. By the late colonial period, *batabs* appealed to *subdelgados* and *juezes españoles* to mediate their disputes with other *cah* leaders, or to express grievances against Spaniards. Nonelite Maya used the same agencies to complain against their own *batab*. While *cah* leaders still administered justice in their communities, *jueces españoles* intervened in cases of disputes,[19] further evidence of the increased Spanish presence in the *cah*.

Economic reforms accelerated Spanish acquisition of Maya land. Free trade reforms within the empire opened the port of Campeche to Spanish ships from the region, stimulating the regional economy. The traditional cattle estates of the northwest expanded with increased demand. So too did the production of henequen. The fiber from henequen plants made fine cordage, especially for ships' rigging. Small-scale production of this product began in the northwest late in the colonial period, but it became increasinly important over the course of the nineteenth century. Sugar production expanded rapidly in the hilly *Puuc* region, the region that separated the drier northwest from the wetter and more forested southern regions. A network of roads sustained commercial relations among the market towns of Tekax, Peto, and Tihosuco.[20] Maya residents satisfied the labor demands for the cattle, henequen, and sugar estates, many of which grew at the expense of *cah* holdings.

Demographic growth compounded the demand for land. Maya populations had recovered over the course of the eighteenth century, even as the Spanish and mestizo population increased. Some 358,000 people occupied Yucatán in 1800, the bulk of them Maya. By 1845, just before the Caste War, that number had increased to 580,000 people.[21]

Yucatán did little to earn its independence from Spain. It became part of the Mexican Republic in 1821, but then declared its independence in 1839, joining in a brief alliance with the Republic of Texas. Though it nominally rejoined the country in 1846, not until Maximilian's Empire was defeated in 1867 were relationships between Yucatán and Mexico "normalized." Yucatán's leaders maintained an attitude of independence from the federal government. This sense of distance from Mexican reality sustains the belief that Yucatán has been a "land apart," different and ignored by central Mexico. Local elite nurtured this nationalist attitude, especially when federal policies might hinder their economic or political priorities.

As had been the case since the early colonial period, Mérida and Campeche vied for regional domination in the years after independence. In 1811, Spanish authorities opened the port of Sisal to international trade, a move that amplified Mérida's position and dramatically lowered the cost of transporting products to the coast. As sugar and the henequen industry developed, exports from Sisal surpassed those of Campeche, reaching twice their value by 1845.[22] Valladolid too profited from the sugar industry, increasing its influence in the eastern portion of the state.

Sugar changed the world of the Maya, leading directly to the Caste War. The government of Yucatán sold public lands to facilitate the growth of sugar estates in an effort to raise money. Most sugar was grown in the corn zone, where Maya communities had used these areas for *milpa* production, producing an economic and social strain upon the region. Moreover, sugar production demanded considerable labor, which the state helped to provide by permitting the debt peonage pattern of northwest Yucatán in the sugar zone. The population of the region boomed, with almost one out of three residents of Yucatán living in the sugar zone by 1847, the year the war began.

Contrary to its popular name, the Caste War was not simply a war between *dzules* and Maya.[23] More broadly, the conflict consisted of two "stages," the first of which pitted whites, Maya, and many mestizos of the east and south against whites, mestizos, and their Maya allies of the west and northwest.[24] Regional struggles among whites in Valladolid, Mérida, and Campeche for control of the state political structure constituted a second stage. Many locate the origin of the conflict to the 1839 revolt of Santiago Imán in eastern Yucatán, a movement that captured Mérida with the assistance of armed Maya rebels. Several years of political struggles among whites exacerbated racial tensions, leading to a "Maya" revolt in 1847. Around 1850, the rebellion took on a religious tone, as the "talking cross" inspired Maya rebels. After Maya seized much of the state, whites reversed the tide of war, establishing a "pacified" region around Mérida. After 1853, with the establishment of white/Maya "peace" accord, white political contestations persisted until 1867. Rebels fled southward, asserting loyalty to the *cruzob* in Chan Santa Cruz. They successfully resisted whites in the southeast until the final outpost of the *cruzob* was conquered by federal troops in 1901.

The Caste War altered the racial and geographic complexion of the region. An 1850 census showed a population loss of over 200,000 people in just four years. Reed estimates that 80,000 people died in the early stages of the war, but more fled the fighting.[25] The southeast region saw the heaviest fighting, leading to significant population losses. Many Maya fled south into more heavily forested regions or into the northwest, whereas whites sought safety in the relative security of the northwest. Whereas the areas around Mérida saw their populations increase by almost fifty percent, populations in the zones with the heaviest fighting fell by a similar amount. Maya population figures did not reach their prewar total until the 1930s.[26]

Social nomenclatures changed dramatically because of the war. The 1853 peace agreement led whites to distinguish "pacified" Indians who had accepted the accord from the "*bravos*" who remained in arms. The regions around Valladolid and south of the *Puuc* housed pacified Maya, while Quintana Roo was the refuge of the *bravos*. Peter Hervick relates that pacified Maya replaced their earlier *masewal* identity with that of mestizos, who might also be called *catrines* or *gente del vestido*, depending upon their degree of acculturation. Rebels continued to refer to themselves as *masewales*. Hervick argues that while *catrines* might wear Western clothes and speak more Spanish, they would not completely reject their Maya heritage. By contrast, *gente de vestido* would leave their villages and accept a new, often urban lifestyle.[27]

The Caste War facilitated the creation of a Maya "other" by Yucatec whites, including those in Mérida's medical community. Founders of Yucatán's first medical society, the *Sociedad Médico-Farmaceutica* (Medical-Pharmaceutical Society, 1871), spoke of residents of the "interior" as barbarians who held secrets unknown to civilized residents.[28] This juxtaposition of civilization and barbarianism symbolized the White mission after the Caste War, and illustrated a pervasive ideology throughout Latin America.[29] Public health programs were both civilizing missions and efforts of control of the barbarous interior. As Heather McCrea relates, this ideology protected "the public from diseases while simultaneously advancing the civilizing mission as a justification for ending the Caste War by any means possible. . . ."[30] Argentines and Bolivians sought to "civilize" indigenous others by similar public health policies.[31]

Henequen and the Modernization of Yucatán

Henequen transformed much of Yucatán; leading to a "*belle epoque*" that lasted from 1880 through the 1910s. At the start of the Caste War, northwest Yucatán was a mixed agricultural zone, in which small farmers, Maya communities, and Spanish haciendas produced corn, cattle, foodstuffs, sugar, and small amounts of henequen. By 1900, haciendas dominated the northwest, with miles and miles of henequen spikes, laboriously worked by debt peons, enslaved Yaquis, and salaried laborers. Henequen enriched a powerful elite—the *casta divina*—who forged potent relations with the regime of Porfirio Díaz, solidified their political influence in the region, and became intimately connected to foreign capital.

The henequen plant thrived in the soils of northwest Yucatán. A member of the *agave* family, the most commonly planted type in the region was *Agave fourcroydes*. Commercial plantings of henequen consisted of long rows that needed careful weeding during their first year of growth. Some five to seven years later, the leaves could be cut, which, given the plant's twenty-year life span, meant that planters could expect some fifteen years of productivity. Leaves were cut on a yearlong basis.

Technology both facilitated the production of henequen fibers and dramatically increased the demand for those fibers. Allen Wells relates that some 500 henequen leaves had to be scraped—by hand—to produce one pound of fiber. It took ten days to free the fibers from the 2,000 leaves cut in one day. The invention of a mechanical rasper in the 1850s—the *decorticator*—allowed each machine to produce some 350 pounds of fiber a day.[32] Concurrently, the development of a mechanical knotting device for the McCormick binder in the 1870s opened the floodgates of demand for binder twine to tie sheaves of wheat. Henequen twine permitted the development of the wheat industry on the plains of the United States and Canada. Eighty-five percent of the binder twine used in North America in 1900 originated in Yucatán.[33]

The prosperity of the postwar henequen industry transformed Yucatán. From one of Mexico's poorest states, it was the wealthiest by 1900. In 1877, at the start of the boom, Mérida numbered some 30,000 residents; by 1910, that number had doubled. By 1890, Yucatán boasted the largest and most extensive rail network in Mexico; 1,600 kilometers of intermediate gauge were used on the haciendas; some 800 kilometers of standard gauge linked the region. Mérida enjoyed its position as the hub of the four major rail lines in the state. Most of these lines were united in the *Ferrocarriles Unidos de Yucatán* in 1902. The new port of Progreso, opened in 1871, served as the terminus of the rail system and the connection to international transportation lines. Warehouses stored the fiber to be shipped from a pier that reached two miles in length by 1939 to accommodate ocean-going vessels.[34]

The henequen industry required extensive credit, most of it from US sources. In the years it took for the spikes to reach maturity, machinery needed to be purchased from abroad; intermediate gauge tramways needed to be built and connected to rail lines; and labor payrolls needed to be met. Low prices forced borrowing. Export houses served as the primary source of credit to the *hacendados*. These houses in turn borrowed from US banks and buyers.

Politics served as a powerful linkage between Yucatán and the federal government of Porfirio Díaz. Díaz's system of *destape*—the presidential selection of state governors—strengthened the federal influence in Yucatán, while forcing the president to respond to the interests of the region's political factions, or *camarillas*. The three political *camarillas* were linked to different export houses, reinforcing the close relationship between henequen wealth and political power. Control of the apparatus of state government enabled *camarillas* to extend their influence throughout the state, often by the appointment of *jefes políticos* of the *partidos* and municipalities, officials who both served as tools for campaigning and repression. Competing *camarillas* sought the support of henequen *hacendados* and members of the merchant class, thereby extending their influence on political decision-making. Small town residents competed for advantages in the political system, with local rivals attaching themselves to one or another *camarilla* as best suited their interests.[35] Patronage networks extended from Mérida into the smallest villages, forging competing "multi-class coalitions" that enlivened electoral politics.[36]

The three *camarillas* vied for the gubernatorial selection of 1898. Pancho Cantón, a regional caudillo from Valladolid, had supported Díaz since the 1876 uprising. The henequen merchant Olegario Molina aspired to the position, as did incumbent governor Peón Machado. A profoundly divisive contest led to Díaz's appointment of Cantón, whose administration witnessed the forced separation of Quintana Roo from Yucatán after the victory over the *cruzob*. Molina's support of this highly unpopular decision by Mexico City, combined with his "scientific" attitudes, resulted in his selection as governor in 1902.[37]

Henequen wealth sharpened an already rigid social hierarchy. Thirty or forty families made wealthy by the production or marketing of the fiber occupied the highest echelon. These *parentescos* (elite family networks) dominated the region's economy and had powerful political influences. Closely linked to them were perhaps 400 families statewide who constituted the elite of the region. Middle sectors tended to be urban, comprised of professionals, small merchants, lawyers, physicians, and the like. Physicians came from both the elite and middle sectors. Urban "working classes" included artisans and wage laborers, many of whom were associated with the henequen industry. Wage laborers were also associated with the system of railroad that webbed the region, workers who would later sustain a potent labor union. The bulk of the rural population, including *campesinos*, henequen *peones*, and *indios del pueblo,* constituted an estimated sixty percent of the state's population. A small foreign-born population also resided in the state, ranging from US merchants associated with the henequen industry, to Lebanese merchants in Mérida, to the Chinese and Korean workers who labored in near slavery on the haciendas. Working under similar restraints were Yaqui Indians whose revolt in Sonora earned them exile in Yucatán.[38] The gap between the top and the bottom of the ladder was enormous, as the comparison between the mansions along *Paseo Montejo* and the Maya *na* (thatched house) vividly demonstrates.

Despite the lifestyles of the *casta divina*, Yucatec society at the beginning of the twentieth century was largely impoverished, rural, and dominated by Maya speakers. Mérida's literacy rate barely passed forty percent; rural Yucatán counted only three in ten who could read. Most people lived in villages of less than 500; only seven towns had more than 4,000 residents, with Valladolid at 12,000 and Mérida at 60,000.[39] The 1900 census reported that 69 percent of the adult population spoke Maya as their birth language. Most rural whites and large numbers of urban whites used the language as well.[40] The state of Yucatán totaled some 340,000 people in 1910, an increase of only 42,000 since 1794. It would boom to 622,243 over the next fifty years. Urbanization and the development of new towns in the eastern and southern portions of the state drove much of the population increase.[41]

THE EMERGENCE OF THE WHITE CITY

A common vision of modernization shaped the transformation of many Latin American cities in the late nineteenth century. With Paris as the model, urban planners constructed wide boulevards, tore down tenement houses to make way for mansions, built opera houses, and undertook water, sewage, and paving projects. Public health agencies sought a more sanitary environment.

Redesigned police forces were only one of the many new mechanisms for social control. "Naturally," the wealthy and the emerging middle sectors were the primary beneficiaries of the modern city, other residents benefited only marginally; many suffered at the expense of modernization.

The *Olegariato* (1901–06) spawned the rapid transformation of Mérida. Governor Molina and regional elites shared a vision of a modernized state and had the money to fund it. Although the transformation of the city had begun in the 1880s, it expanded dramatically under Molina. Wells and Joseph relate how Molina "coaxed" funds from the henequen elite to help underwrite the construction of a new Hospital O'Horán, the *Asilo Ayala* for the mentally ill, and the Juárez penitentiary in a zone about two kilometers from the city's center. The dazzling Peón Contreras Theater went up a block from the *Plaza de Armas*. Downtown streets were paved, a drainage system was installed, and the town square refurbished. A new marketplace was built several blocks from the plaza. Tram lines were expanded, especially toward the north and west. Surrounding the center, the plazas of several barrios were refurbished to include markets, police stations, offices, stores, and new churches. The highlight of the transformative enterprise was the creation of the tree-lined *Paseo Montejo* to the north of the center, along which elites built enormous mansions.[42] Mérida had become the "white city."[43]

Not surprisingly, the Molina *parentesco* benefited directly from these urban projects. O. Molina y Compañia shared the drainage and paving project with the Philadelphia-based Mérida Water Company. Family members occupied key positions in the state. One of Olegario's brothers served as president of the board of United Railroads of Yucatán; another—Augusto Molina Solís—served as Director of the School of Medicine and held a seat in the congress; another Olegario's son-in-law was the local agent for International Harvester and held multiple public and private posts; one nephew was the *jefe político* of Mérida; and another—Ignacio Molina Castilla—occupied a key position at the Hospital O'Horán. The list could continue. In part not only due to his relationship with International Harvester, but also due to his adept use of political power, Olegario Molina became the largest landowner in the state and the largest single producer of henequen.[44]

The *Olegariato* evoked considerable dissent. Political opponents were harassed, arrested, and often housed in the new penitentiary. A nascent labor movement grew among workers created by the henequen boom, including workers at the docks and from the rail system. Elite opposition forces strengthened after Molina was re elected in 1906. When Díaz tapped Molina as federal secretary of development, his replacement's repressive tactics worsened the situation. The Cantón *camarilla* strengthened as henequen prices fell with the 1907 economic panic, whereas many professionals sought avenues of political reform. Urban labor and rural workers strengthened their organizations, displaying more militancy in the wake of Madero's uprising. Still, though the calm of the region was upset, it did not join in the revolutionary movement of the 1910s.[45]

THE BIOMEDICAL TRANSFORMATION

Over the course of the nineteenth century, biomedicine became a scientific belief system supported by a range of institutions and state policies. Differences between domestic, national, and international understandings of these new medical practices were small, though innovations tended to emerge from what became biomedical centers. These biomedical centers were typically located in Western Europe, joined in time by the United States. Advocates and practitioners of biomedicine constituted a larger Atlantic medical community, in which Yucatec physicians actively participated. The region's medical institutions illustrate Yucatán's position in the emerging Atlantic biomedical community.

The *Escuela de Medicina* in Mérida, founded in 1833, offered training to Yucatec physicians. Its curriculum paralleled the emerging biomedical field, with a relationship with the General Hospital and, after 1906, a strong emphasis on laboratory science. Though a smattering of Yucatec physicians received their education abroad or migrated to the region, most physicians were educated locally.

Direct international influences in the development of the Yucatec public health system were limited, though their general influence grew over time. Technologies such as smallpox vaccine were part of the public health mission, as were changes in medical education. The sanitation movement shaped the function of the *Junta Superior de Sanidad*, as did general tendencies within the international community regarding diseases such as yellow fever. Yucatec officials were conversant in methods of attacking yellow fever and other diseases, even while knowledge and techniques originated outside the state and region. The region was certainly not a center of innovation, but it participated in the national and international conversations. However, political and public health officials took steps to achieve their domestic objectives, centering public health policy in Mérida.

The construction of a "modern" public health infrastructure proceeded rapidly in the first years of the twentieth century. Buoyed by ample funds derived from the henequen economy, and sustained by an elite "Chilango blueprint" for modernization, medical institutions in 1920 bore little resemblance to those of the nineteenth century. The creation of a permanent public health board in 1894, the 1906 construction of the 400-bed Hospital O'Horán, and the professionalization of the state's biomedical corps constitute key steps in the modernization project. Gradually at first, but with a rapid acceleration, biomedical facilities sustained the transformation of Yucatán's medical system.

The 1894 creation of a permanent public health agency constituted the foundation of the biomedical project. The *Junta Superior de Sanidad* responded not only to long-standing local demands, but also to clauses in the Federal Sanitary Code in 1891 urging states to create such organizations. The *Junta Superior de Sanidad* encompassed a broad range of "modern" public health concerns, many of them reflective of the sanitarian movement.[46] The capital's team consisted of several *vocales* with responsibilities for different sections of the city. Each representative managed the *Junta*'s activities in the sections, responded to cases of infectious diseases, inspected prostitutes, and conducted basic sanitary inspections. The *Junta* had a small delegation in Progreso with limited facilities.[47] A major reorganization in 1917 focused upon laboratory facilities to test the quality of milk, drugs, and other products. During a smallpox epidemic in 1915 and the influenza outbreak of 1918–19, the *Junta Superior* organized Auxiliary Health Units in provincial towns to combat localized outbreaks of the disease. These came to be the mainstay of the public health system in the countryside. Still, the *Junta Superior* did very little to extend its influence into the henequen or corn zones of the state, leaving the vast majority of citizens without access to formal health care.

The Hospital O'Horán adhered to the model of the modern hospital established by the earlier reorganization of Johns Hopkins University. This system linked a hospital, medical school, clinics, and laboratories. Physicians associated with the School of Medicine and Hospital O'Horán used the hospital's clinics and laboratories to experiment with new medical procedures. A new chair of psychiatry produced interns for the Asilo Ayla.[48] Danish-born Harald Seidilin created a "museum of pathological anatomy" so that he and his associates could utilize the dead for teaching purposes and the investigation of disease.[49]

The federal government had an extremely limited role in Yucatec public health, with most attention paid to yellow fever. Convinced by the success of the US program against yellow fever in Havana, Mexico launched a nationwide campaign against the disease in 1903. At first, Yucatec officials declined to cooperate with the federal delegates, as the governor insisted that the federal government had no right to intrude upon the state's jurisdiction, and that the state would have no financial obligation in supporting the campaign.[50] The relationship between state and federal officials gradually improved, though funding remained a flash point. As federal delegates withdrew from the region at the start of the Revolution, local physician Gil Rojas Aguilar assumed the responsibility as the federal sanitary delegate in Mérida. In 1914, the Federal Anti-Yellow Fever Service (*Servicio Federal contra la Fiebre Amarilla*) was placed under the jurisdiction of the *Junta Superior*.[51]

The Mexican Revolution spawned the reconceptualization of the federal health mission. In the 1920s, the federal government expanded the functions of its sanitary delegation in Yucatán, seeking a more autonomous role in the region. Revolutionary federal officials used biomedicine to modernize and civilize rural dwellers, whose traditional medical practices allegedly "hindered" the progress of the nation.[52] Federal and state officials endorsed the civilizing function of public health, seeking to impart "scientific" notions among the "ignorant, superstitious" villagers and their "witch doctors."[53] Federal officials asserted in the 1940s that problems with indigenous peoples were fundamentally cultural, "so that it was necessary to integrate them into the rest of the Mexican society."[54]

Yucatán's henequen estates symbolized one of the strongest pre revolutionary power bases in the nation. As Lázaro Cárdenas declared rural public health to be part of the six-year plan of his presidency, he faced an enormous obstacle in the power of the henequen elite. Cárdenas announced the nationalization of henequen *ejidos* in 1937, declaring that health care programs modeled after those of Michoacán and Nuevo León would be part of the newly created henequen *ejidos*. While the local elite could not block the land seizures, they dominated the *Henequeneros de Yucatán*, a locally controlled organization that oversaw the sale of henequen in overseas markets and thereby insured their continued profits of the industry. Still, revolutionary health care objectives were satisfied with the creation of a "social assistance" program for henequen *ejidos*, following the federal model, but managed by state public health officials.[55] By the late 1940s, the social assistance program of the *Henequeneros* included a major hospital in Mérida, over seventy rural dispensaries, and eleven mobile health units.

Federal sanitary delegates undertook several initiatives throughout the state beginning in the 1930s, notably campaigns against tuberculosis, venereal disease, and malaria. The most significant federal successes lay in extending public health into the Yucatec corn zone. Federal "*servicios de higiene rural y medicina social*" (Rural Hygiene and Social Medicine Services) began in 1936. Both henequen and corn *ejido* members paid at least half of the cost of health services, which included health education, food inspections, and inoculations against communicable diseases.[56] Irwin Press describes how these agencies became important medical fixtures in the corn zone, helping to inculcate biomedical beliefs among younger residents.[57]

The decline of henequen prices after 1945 led to the collapse of the *Henequeneros de Yucatán*. The federal government assumed control of both the henequen distribution network and the medical facilities of the zone in 1955. In 1958, Yucatán's henequen *ejidos* had the most complex medical facilities of any region in the country. Eight separate medical zones divided the henequen zone, each of which boasted a small hospital, multiple sanitary units, and multiple first aid stations. In Mérida, the 400 bed *Hospital 20 de Noviembre* offered the widest range of medical care in the state.[58] By the late 1950s, health clinics in both the corn and henequen zones became part of the national health network of the *Secretaría de Salubridad y Asistencia.*

The development of a biomedical public health system altered Yucatec society in many ways. Public health officials achieved considerable social and political prestige as biopower expanded with the growth of the state. Their sanitation codes intruded upon childbirth, illness, and death, making the state an actor in key moments of life. Codes affected a myriad of other parts of day-to-day life, including drinking water, the cleanliness of streets, or upon how to construct one's home.[59] In time, biomedicine changed the nature of disease in the peninsula, as well as how people responded to illnesses. Biomedicine and the public health project proved to be a potent source of state power, one that no doubt satisfied the modernizing objectives of its proponents.

NOTES

1. Servicios Sanitarios Coordinadores, Enfermedades Transmisibles to the Auditor General of the Departamento de Beneficencia y Sanidad, November 27, 1939, Archivo General del Estado de Yucatán (hereafter AGEY), Sección Junta Superior de Sanidad (JSS), Series Copiador de Oficios, Volume 190, No. 1384.

2. *Memoria de la Secretaría de Salubridad y Asistencia Pública. Sexenio 1952–1958* (México DF: Impreso for ACMEX, S. A., 1958), 520, 528.

3. Allen Wells and Gilbert Joseph, "Modernizing Visions, Chilango Blueprints, and Provincial Growing Pains: Mérida at the Turn of the Century," *Mexican Studies/Estudios Mexicanos* 8:2 (Summer 1992), 167–215.

4. Matthew Restall, *The Black Middle: Africans, Mayas, and Spaniards in Colonial Yucatán* (Stanford: Stanford University Press, 2009).

5. Matthew Restall, *The Maya World: Yucatec Culture and Society, 1550–1850* (Stanford: Stanford University Press, 1997), 18; Peter Hervik, *Mayan People Within and Beyond Boundaries: Social Categories and Lived Identity in Yucatán* (Amsterdam: Harwood Academic Publishers, 1999), 36–42.

6. Grant D. Jones, *Maya Resistance to Spanish Rule: Time and History on a Colonial Frontier* (Albuquerque: University of New Mexico Press, 1989), 10–11.

7. Inga Clendinnen, *Ambivalent Conquests: Maya and Spaniard in Yucatán,* 1517–1570 (New York: Cambridge University Press, 1987), 42.

8. Nancy M. Farriss, *Maya Society under Colonial Rule: the Collective Enterprise of Survival* (Princeton: Princeton University Press, 1984), 52–56; Jeffery Brannon and Eric N. Baklanoff, *Agrarian Reform and Public Enterprise in Mexico: The Political Economy of Yucatán's Henequen Industry* (Tuscaloosa: The University of Alabama Press, 1987), 21–22.

9. Pedro Bracamonte y Sosa and Gabriela Solís Robleda, *Espacios Mayas de autónomia: el pacto colonial en Yucatán* (Mérida: Universidad Autónoma de Yucatán, 1996), 13.

10. Bracamonte y Sosa and Solís Robleda, *El pacto colonial*, 43–49, 60–74.

11. Restall, *The Maya World*, 13–40, 51–60.

12. Sherburne F. Cook and Woodrow Borah, "The Population of Yucatán, 1517–1960," in *Essays in Population History: Mexico and the Caribbean*, 3 vols. (Berkeley: University of California Press, 1974), Vol. 2, 75, 79, 85–86, 94, 114.

13. Robert Patch, *Maya and Spaniard in Yucatán, 1648–1812* (Stanford: Stanford University Press, 1994), 42–44.

14. Patch, *Maya and Spaniard*, 43.

15. Marco Antonio Palma Solís, *La educación médica en Yucatán* (Mérida: Universidad Autónoma de Yucatán, 1990), 60–61.

16. Mariana Appel Kunow, *Maya Medicine: Traditional Healing in Yucatán* (Albuquerque: University of New Mexico Press, 2003), 9–10; Munro S. Edmonson and Victoria R. Bricker, "Yucatecan Mayan Literature," in *Supplement to the Handbook of Middle American Indians, Volume Three, Literatures*, ed. by Munro S. Edmonson (Austin: University of Texas Press, 1985), 45, 52; Ralph L. Roys, *The Ethno-Botany of the Maya* (New Orleans: Tulane University, 1931. Republished by ISHI Reprints on Latin America and the Caribbean. Philadelphia, 1976), xix.

17. For a political overview of this period, see Melchor Campos García, *De provincia a estado de la república Mexicana: La península de Yucatán, 1786–1835* (Mérida: Universidad Autónoma de Yucatán, Consejo Nacional de Ciencia y Tecnología, 2004).

18. Bracamonte y Sosa and Solís Robleda, *El pacto colonial*, 54.

19. Farriss, *Maya Society under Colonial Rule*, 356–59.

20. Allen Wells, *Yucatán's Gilded Age: Haciendas, Henequen, and International Harvester, 1860–1915* (Albuquerque: University of New Mexico Press, 1985), 23.

21. Cook and Borah, "The Population of Yucatán," 123–24; Nelson A. Reed, *The Caste War of Yucatán*, rev. ed. (Stanford: Stanford University Press, 2001), 5.

22. Brannon and Baklanoff, *Agrarian Reform and Public Enterprise in Mexico*, 24.

23. Many people have written on the Caste War. See as leading examples, Moisés González Navarro, *Raza y tierra: La guerra de castas y el henequén* (México DF: El Colegio de México, 1970); Reed, *The Caste War of Yucatán*; Terry Rugeley, *Yucatán's Maya Peasantry and the Origins of the Caste War* (Austin: University of Texas Press, 1996); Rugely, *Rebellion Now and Forever: Mayas, Hispanics, and Caste War Violence in Yucatán,* 1800–1880 (Stanford: Stanford University Press, 2009); Don E. Dumond, *The Machete and the Cross: Campesino Rebellion in Yucatán* (Lincoln: University of Nebraska Press, 1997).

24. Hervik, *Mayan People Within and Beyond Boundaries*, 42–43.

25. Reed, *The Caste War of Yucatán*, 141–42.

26. Cook and Borah, "The Population of Yucatán," 128–29.

27. Hervik, *Mayan People Within and Beyond Boundaries*, 43–50. This distinction might be specific to the Puuc town of Oxkutzcab, where he studied; the many case studies of Yucatán reveal that the diversity of the region undermines the concept of a homogeneous Maya experience.

28. *La Emulación*, February 1873.

29. Domingo Sarmiento, *Facundo: Civilization and Barbarism*, translated by Roberto Eche Varría González and Kathleen Ross (Berkeley: University of California

Press, 2003); Brooke Larson, *Trials of Nation Making: Liberalism, Race, and Ethnicity in the Andes,* 1810–1910 (New York: Cambridge University Press, 2004).

30. McCrea, *Diseased Relations*, 96.

31. See, for example, Julia Rodríguez, *Civilizing Argentina: Science, Medicine, and the Modern State* (Chapel Hill: The University of North Carolina Press, 2006); Ann Zulawaski, *Unequal Cures: Public Health and Political Change in Bolivia, 1900–1950* (Duke University Press, 2007).

32. Brannon and Baklanoff, *Agrarian Reform and Public Enterprise in Mexico*, 37.

33. Wells, *Gilded Age*, 28; Brannon and Baklanoff, *Agrarian Reform and Public Enterprise in Mexico*, 37.

34. Wells and Joseph, *Summer of Discontent*, 127–29; Brannon and Baklanoff, *Agrarian Reform and Public Enterprise in Mexico*, 38; Henry A. Case, *Views on and of Yucatán Besides Notes upon parts of the state of Campeche and the Territory of Quintana Roo* (Mérida: Henry A. Case, 1911), 9.

35. Paul Eiss, *In the Name of the Pueblo: Place, Community, and the Politics of History in Yucatán* (Durham: Duke University Press, 2010).

36. This section relies heavily upon Wells and Joseph, *Summer of Discontent, Seasons of Upheaval*, 21–31.

37. Wells and Joseph, *Summer of Discontent,* 32–43, 51–52, 63, 64.

38. Marisa Pérez de Sarmiento and Franco Savarino Roggero, *El cultivo de las élites. Grupos económicos y politicos en Yucatán en los siglos XIX y XX* (México DF: Conaculta, 2001), 115; Asael T. Hansen, "Change in the Class System of Mérida, Yucatán, 1875–1935," in *Yucatán: A World Apart*, ed. by Edward H. Mosely and Edward D. Terry (University, AL: The University of Alabama Press, 1980), 122–41.

39. Brannon and Baklanoff, *Agrarian Reform and Public Enterprise in Mexico*, 40; Cook and Borah, "The Population of Yucatán."

40. Pérez de Sarmiento and Savarino Roggero, *El cultivo de las élites*, 112.

41. Cook and Borah, "The Population of Yucatán," 153, 174.

42. Molina also reorganized the police force and created a secret police to assist in maintaining order in the region. Wells and Joseph, *Summer of Discontent*, 69–70. On the transformation of the city, see Wells and Joseph, "Modernizing Visions"; José Humberto Fuentes Gómez and Magnolia Rosado Lugo, "Mérida: La obra urbana en el porfiriato," in *Identidades sociales en Yucatán*, compiled by María Cecilia Lara Cebada (Mérida: Universidad Autónoma de Yucatán, Facultad de Ciencias Antropológicas, 1997), 71–98; Asael T. Hansen and Juan R. Bastarrachea M., *Mérida; Su transformación: de capital colonial a naciente metrópolis* (Mexico: Instituto Nacional de Antropología e Historia, 1984).

43. Enrique Urzaiz Lares, "La arquitectura Porfiriana en Mérida," in *Mérida: El azar y la memoria*, Marco Tulio Peraza Guzmán et al. (Mérida: Asociación de Personal Académico, Universidad Autónoma de Yucatán, 1993), 89–114.

44. Wells and Joseph, *Summer of Discontent*, 64–65, 98–99,131.

45. Wells and Joseph, *Summer of Discontent*, 64, 65–70, 89–92.

46. *Boletín de Higiene*, May 5, 1895.

47. Joaquín Patrón and Agustín Cáceres to the President of the Consejo Superior de Salubridad de México, February 5, 1903, Mérida, Archivo General del Estado de

Yucatán (AGEY), Fondo Poder Ejecutivo (FPE), Sección Junta Superior de Sanidad (JSS), Serie Copiador de Oficios, Volume 11, entry 5951.

48. "Sintesis biográfica Dr. Eduardo Urzaiz Rodríguez," Archivo Histórico de la Educación en Yucatán, Fondo Maestros Distinguidos, Expediente Materiales Mixtas, Eduardo Urzaiz Rodríguez; *La Revista Médica de Yucatán*, November 1908.

49. *La Revista Médica de Yucatán*, February 1910.

50. Francisco Cárdenas to Eduardo Liceaga, Mérida, December 31, 1906, Archivo Histórico de la Secretaría de Salubridad y Asistencia (ASSHA), Fondo Salud Pública (FSP), Sección Epidemiologia, Caja 5, exp. 5; Enrique Múñoz Arístequi to Liceaga, February 4, April 17, June 12, June 19, 1907 ibid.; Liceaga to Múñoz, Mexico City, April 24, 1907, May 13, 1907, ibid.

51. Secretary of the Departamento de Salubridad Pública to Jefe de Hacienda of the state of Yucatán, Mexico City, July 26, 1922, ASSHA, FSP, Sección Epidemiología, Caja 30, exp. 10.

52. Gilbert M. Joseph and Daniel Nugent, eds., *Everyday Forms of State Formation: Revolution and the Negotiation of Rule in Modern Mexico* (Durham: Duke University Press, 1994); James Horn, "The Mexican Revolution and Health Care or the Health of the Mexican Revolution," *International Journal of Health Services* 15:3 (1985), 485–99; Heather McCrea, *Diseased Relations*; Ben Fallaw, *Cárdenas Compromised: The Failure of Reform in Postrevolutionary Yucatán* (Durham, NC: Duke University Press, 2001).

53. Gordon Schendel, *Medicine in Mexico* (Austin: University of Texas Press, 1968).

54. Hector Hernández Llamas, "La atención médica en el medio rural mexicano," in Hector Hernández Llamas, compiler, *La atención médica rural en México, 1930–1980* (México DF: Instituto Mexicano de Seguro Social, 1984), 28.

55. *Informe del Sr. Ingeniero Humberto Canto E., Gobernador Constitucional de Yucatán ante la XXIV legislatura del estado 1939* (Mérida: Imprenta del Estado, 1940).

56. Dirección de Servicios Sanitarios Coordinados en los Estados y Territorios, *Directorio General, 1940*, April 2, 1940, Archivo General de la Nación (AGN), Fondo Lázaro Cárdenas del Río (LCR), Caja 185, 425.5/179.

57. Irwin Press, *Tradition and Adaptation: Life in a Modern Yucatán Maya Village* (Westport, CT: Greenwood Press, 1975).

58. *Memoria* 1952–1958, 530–35.

59. Cueto, *The Value of Heath*, 28–29; Foucault, *The History of Sexuality: An Introduction, Volume 1* (New York: Random House, 1990).

Chapter 2

Institutionalizing Biomedicine

The medical complex surrounding the Hospital O'Horán is still impressive over 100 years after its construction. Occupying almost ninety acres of land on the outskirts of Mérida, it included over 40 isolated wings for patient care, several specialized hospital and laboratory facilities, and physicians who worked intimately with the School of Medicine to institute "modern" medical practices into the facility. President Porfirio Díaz made his first visit to the state to dedicate the Hospital O'Horán and its companion Asylum Ayala on February 6, 1906, symbolizing the unity between Yucatec modernizers and the vision of the Porfiriato.[1] Hospital O'Horán illustrated the emergence of a state that would use public health to penetrate the quotidian lives of its citizens, a potent weapon in state formation and the institutionalization of biomedicine in Yucatán.

The hospital was only one facet of what might be seen as a "biomedical plexus,"[2] a unified network of facilities, organizations, physicians, knowledge, and actions that constituted the infrastructure of biomedicine in Yucatán. The *Junta Superior de Sanidad* served as the critical foundation of the plexus; it was responsible for a wide range of activities including sanitary inspections, public health campaigns, and the expansion of "modern" health practices after the 1890s. Prior to the 1930s, the *Junta Superior* acted with limited federal influence, largely in the region of Mérida and the port of Progreso. After the 1930s, revolutionary initiatives from the central government gradually came to dominate the region, with the influence of both state and federal agencies felt statewide. By the 1950s, Yucatán's network of hospitals, clinics, medical corps, and political affiliations sustained one of Mexico's most developed public health systems.

This chapter concentrates on medical institutions associated with the emerging biomedical system. The turn-of-the-century modernization effort divides the chapter into two broad sections. The initial section discusses nineteenth-century public health initiatives, which grew in reaction to smallpox and cholera, diseases that forced physicians and politicians to act—albeit temporarily—in the public interest. The nineteenth century also saw the establishment of a School of Medicine, General Hospital, and the initial "professionalization" of titled physicians. The second section focuses upon two eras of twentieth-century medical institutions, one defined by Yucatec public health initiatives (1894–1930s) and the second by the impact of federal revolutionary projects upon Yucatec institutions (1930s–1950s). Actions taken by public health institutions are discussed in both periods. Throughout, medical schools, hospitals, and physicians were linked in the pursuit of the "progress and civilization" represented by the institutionalization of "modern, scientific" medicine in the daily lives of Yucatec residents.

DISEASE AND THE INSTITUTIONALIZATION OF PUBLIC HEALTH

Disease played a profound role in the development of Yucatán's nineteenth-century public health institutions. Small pox had plagued the peninsula since the conquest period; Edward Jenner's 1796 development of a vaccine offered hope for a means to fight that deadly disease. Local officials sought out the vaccine to undertake their own vaccination programs, as did physicians in many areas of the Atlantic world. Surprisingly, the Spanish government undertook a bold campaign to immunize subjects throughout its vast empire. The Philantropic Vaccination Campaign (*Expedición Filantrópica de la Vacuna*, 1803–13) has been described by Catherine Mark and José G. Rigau-Pérez as the "world's first immunization campaign," in that it joined clinical, administrative, epidemiologic, and ethical features.[3] Francisco Xavier de Balmis led the expedition into the Caribbean, with the goals of vaccinating the general population, training local officials, and establishing vaccination boards to administer the campaign after the expedition left the area.[4] In short, Balmis sought to create a public health network centered on vaccination against smallpox.

Public health patterns set in motion by the Balmis expedition persisted through the nineteenth century. The expedition reached the Yucatec port of Sisal in late 1804, leading to the creation of "Provincial Vaccination Boards" in Mérida, Campeche, and Valladolid to develop and administer the vaccine.[5] The expedition stayed in Yucatán for only a few weeks before traveling on to Mexico City, where some 100,000 persons were inoculated. Vice-regal officials took charge of the campaign, which survived the turbulence of the struggle for independence.[6]

The anti-smallpox campaign illustrates the troubled relationship between the Yucatec and Mexican governments, and the obstacles in building a public health infrastructure. Tensions lay in part over the production and distribution of vaccine. Federal public health officials directed the campaign, including the production of the vaccine for distribution to state officials, which generally fell short of Yucatec needs. Mérida's municipal council and the governor coordinated smallpox vaccination efforts in the state through the *Dirección General de Vacuna* (General Vaccination Directory).[7] They would appoint "vaccinators" in small towns, using the town council, *jefes políticos*, or clerics as local managers. State officials repeatedly requested more vaccine from the federal government (usually without success), and sought alternative sources.[8] Yucatec officials slowly created a state-wide vaccination system headed by municipal councils and managed by officials in Mérida, even though it lacked reliable sources of vaccine and vaccinators.

While smallpox was all too familiar to the region, the brutal disease that struck Mérida in 1833 was completely unknown. After years of isolation in the Indian subcontinent, cholera appeared in Europe in 1817 and crossed the Atlantic in 1831. It afflicted Yucatán in 1833, coinciding with the emergence of two "first generation" medical leaders. Tomás Antonio O'Horán y Argüello (1775–1848), a lawyer and active politician, had been born in Yucatán, but spent time in Guatemala as a member of the Executive Council of the ill-fated Central American republic. There he met Ignacio Vado Lugo, who was studying for a medical degree, and whom O'Horán urged to further his studies in Paris. After his second degree, Vado Lugo arrived in Sisal in February 1833, where O'Horán invited him to Mérida. Together they sought and gained permission to found an *Escuela de Medicina*, which was chartered in June, days before cholera arrived in the region.[9]

The disease struck Campeche in late June, and then rapidly spread throughout the peninsula. The state government responded by the creation of a statewide "*Suprema Junta de Sanidad*" (Supreme Board of Health) under the direction of the governor. Municipal authorities founded emergency health councils in the principal towns of the region, Mérida, Valladolid, Izamal, Tekax, Motul, and Tizimín. Physicians who had yet to begin their teaching responsibilities at the school mobilized to fight the epidemic. Mérida was divided into four wards, each led by a member of the faculty, and each equipped with an emergency room. Isolation served as the primary response to the debilitating illness. Fortunately the epidemic died down after only two months.[10] The public health agencies created for the emergency ceased operations, a typical nineteenth-century pattern.

The *Escuela de Medicina* quickly became the backbone of Yucatán's medical infrastructure. The curriculum adhered to models found throughout Latin America. Students were taught by "Prima" and "Visperas" chairs, with a curriculum focusing upon anatomy, botany, physiology, pathologies, and medical techniques. Students undertook a four-year program to earn their bachelors; two years of clinical experience to earn their *licenciado*; and a medical title could be awarded after another three years. Separate tracks trained surgeons and pharmacists. Half a dozen students had graduated by 1848.[11]

Groups supporting the School of Medicine also improved hospital facilities. In 1821, two colonial institutions associated with the Church—the hospital of the Order San Juan de Dios and the Franciscan *Iglesia de la Mejorado*—merged into the *Hospital General de Mérida.*[12] The state government took charge of the facility shortly before the start of the first cholera epidemic. The small facility, with fewer than sixty beds, proved inadequate for the epidemic. In the years that followed, it became the site for the development of clinical and practical skills for students at the School of Medicine, a linkage between hospital and education that was increasingly common in the Atlantic medical community.[13]

Cholera returned to Yucatán in September 1853. Physicians were no more knowledgeable of its cause than twenty years earlier, continuing to believe in a miasmic origin, and lacking an effective therapeutic response. The governor ordered the creation of an emergency *Junta Suprema de Sanidad del Estado* in January, led by a team of six citizens, including Dr. Enrique Pérez Calzadilla, Alejandro MacKinsey, José María Tappan, Joaquín Muñoz, José María Domínguez, and Nemesio de los Santos Rubio y Palomeque.[14] Medical students again assisted faculty in alleviating the populace's misery, as did priests in many rural communities. Many died tending to the ill, including Dr. Vado Lugo in October of 1853. The heavy loss of life from the two-year epidemic compounded the misery and social strife from the Caste War, which had displaced thousands of residents away from zones of conflict. Concentrated water supplies—either from wells or *cenotes* (water-filled sinkholes)—amplified the effects of the disease, furthering the population displacement caused by the war.

The rapid onset of cholera—large numbers of people died six to ten hours after the initial symptoms of the disease—and loss of life overwhelmed the capacity of communities to bury the dead. This contributed to political and religious conflict over Yucatán's cemeteries. Heather McCrea notes that liberal efforts to limit the power of the church and to expand state authority led physicians to seek control of burial practices. The numerous deaths from cholera and the speed at which it killed challenged church and cemetery officials. Yucatec tradition dictated a prompt burial, but physicians sought to delay internment in order to verify the cause of death. Liberals from central Mexico used the epidemic as a weapon in their secularization struggle, going so far as to legislate civil burial in 1857. Though the confrontation was less intense in Yucatán,[15] there is evidence of a growing desire among physicians to extend the influence of their profession, even to the grave.

The professionalization of Yucatán's medical corps complemented the construction of a medical infrastructure. Scientific interests and the desire to amplify the influence of biomedical physicians led to the establishment of "*La Sociedad Médico-Farmaceutica*" (The Medical-Pharmaceutical Society) in January 1872.[16] Members insisted upon the need for a permanent public health agency, asserting that "civilized countries" were sustained by public health programs.[17] They also sought to stimulate the study of pharmaceutical and medical practices, forming commissions to study the geography and botany of the region, to gather demographic and medical statistics, and to investigate public health conditions, such as the quality of water and marketplaces as sources of poor sanitation.[18]

The Society argued that reliable medical statistics were necessary for medical progress. It complained that the number of births and deaths in the community were unknown due to the laziness of physicians and the influence of *curanderos* (lay healers). Reliable statistics on deaths could be obtained if the *jefes politicos*—who were in charge of cemeteries—would demand a death certificate before interring a victim.[19] (Twenty years later the permanent Board of Health renewed the campaign for mandatory death certificates—once again with limited success.[20])

Members of the Society defined themselves in juxtaposition to other healing practitioners. Addressing the body in 1873, Waldemaro G. Cantón located healers within a racial and professional context. The labeling of healers as "*charlatanes*," "*curanderos*," "*yerbaleros*," and "*médicos*" (charlatans, healers, herbalists, and doctors) associated race with certain patterns of knowledge, as well as with distinct approaches to healing. The term *médicos* implied university-trained white healers; *yerbaleros* referenced indigenous herbalists who utilized Mayan conceptions of diseases and healings; *curanderos* were lay healers (either indigenous or *mestizo*) who lacked professional training at institutions such as the *Escuela de Medicina*; and charlatans were those healers who practiced without a license or who claimed abilities that they lacked. In his appeal, Cantón admitted that he and other physicians faced serious competition from "charlatans" and "herbalists" if they sought to control medical practices in the region.[21]

The case of José Aké illustrated to the Society the need for fully authorized professional physicians. Aké, a *curandero*, was called to a hacienda to treat the ulcerated leg of an Indian. The healer called the victim's family to the healing ceremony, vaccinating each of them with the pus from the man's leg. All were infected by the inoculation, two of them mortally. Ceferino Monforte, the local magistrate, arrested Aké. The local judge ordered the bodies exhumed and examined by an untitled Cuban physician and two local lay surgeons (*barberos*). Their findings—that the victims died from respiratory infections caused by the injections—were accepted by the judge. Drs. Leocadio Lara and Domingo Avila, titled physicians from Motul, verified the autopsies, but rejected the laymen's findings. Lara and Avila concluded the autopsies did not follow scientific procedures, nor were their conclusions valid insofar as the bodies had been contaminated after death.[22]

Why didn't the judge seek the assistance of titled physicians in the first place? For the Society, the answer was clear; political authorities "not only tolerated the illegal exercise of medicine, they were in fact accomplices of the scandalous intruders (*intrusos*)." The Society insisted that the governor mandate that Legal Medicine (forensics) be the sole responsibility of titled physicians, and that they should refuse to verify the work of non professionals. Legal authority and professional solidarity were both necessary to prevent the "conquest of science by ignorance."[23]

A wave of young physicians transformed the functions of the Hospital General in the second half of the nineteenth century. This generation, many of who were educated abroad, introduced new surgical and medical techniques into the region, often only a few years after their development. José María Tappan, Agustín Jorge O'Horán y Escudero, Luis F. Urcelay Martínez, and Saturnino Guzmán Cervera are often cited as representative of this new generation. O'Horán, the son of independence leader General Tomás O'Horán, graduated from the *Escuela de Medicina* in 1855 and served as director of the hospital from the 1860s until his death in 1884. Tappan, who was born in Philadelphia and educated at Harvard, came to Yucatán in 1846 where he was promptly appointed to the faculty of medicine in obstetrics, a position that he held for almost sixty years. Guzmán Cervera, a graduate of the Medical School in Mérida, went to Paris in 1887 for further study. He returned to Yucatán several years later to perform the first laparoscopy in 1895 and to assume the responsibility for the training of many physicians who would practice in the early twentieth century.[24]

The linkage between the medical school and the hospital matured over the course of the century. Departments of medicine and surgery divided the hospital in 1869, which also operated a *boticario* (pharmacy). Admission to the facility came through the recommendation of its president, Nicolas Almeida, or by a ticket issued by an appropriate political authority. Patients were separated by sex, and might be placed in either the wing for the "sick" or for the "demented."[25] Augusto Molina Solís twice headed both the hospital and the School of Medicine and would play a key role in the establishment of the *Junta Superior de Sanidad*.[26] The General Hospital was renamed as the Hospital O'Horán in 1895, after the death of Agustín Jorge O'Horán Escudero, a name it bears to this date.

MODERN MEDICAL INSTITUTIONS, 1894–1930s

Three institutions serve as foundations for Yucatán's "modern" public health infrastructure—the *Junta Superior de Sanidad*, the hospital complex, and professional medical associations. The critical cornerstone was the *Junta Superior de Sanidad*. The 1906 opening of the Hospital O'Horán medical complex signaled the linkage between medical clinics and medical education. Physicians came together to create a variety of medical organizations, most notably the *Sociedad Médica Yucateca* (Yucatec Medical Society). The interactions of these institutions established the basic of Yucatán's twentieth-century public health system, modified only in the 1930s by the introduction of federally inspired health care clinics in the newly established henequen and corn *ejidos*.

The *Junta Superior de Sanidad* responded not only to long-standing local demands for a permanent board of health, but also to clauses in the Federal Sanitary Code in 1891 that urged states to create such organizations. The *Junta Superior de Sanidad* reported to the governor and was subject to his authority. It had a broad range of responsibilities, including traditional tasks such as responding to epidemics and the management of the smallpox vaccination program. The *Junta* also encompassed a broad range of "modern" public health concerns, many of them reflective of the sanitarian movement. Separate commissions managed Hygiene and Public Sanitation; the practices of medicine and pharmacy; epidemiology, bacteriology, vaccination, medical statistics, and sanitary inspection.[27] The epidemiological and sanitary inspection labors of the body were the most visible to the public.

The smallpox vaccination campaign received increased support with the creation of the *Junta Superior*. In 1889, the state government mandated that all residents be vaccinated, but a shortage of vaccine and vaccinators frustrated that objective.[28] The Vaccination Board maintained regular contact with vaccinators in local towns. Typical of the management effort was a July 1891 note to the *jefe político* of Ticul asking for a list of those who had been vaccinated, and an estimate of how many tubes of vaccine would be needed to complete the task.[29] The campaign became somewhat easier with the establishment of the *Junta Superior*, as it could appoint physicians to replace poorly trained vaccinators. Few doctors wished to take positions outside the capital however. An outbreak in 1897 revealed the need to redouble the efforts of the *Junta Superior*. Between 1893 and 1907 over 256,000 people were vaccinated, perhaps three-quarters of the state's population.[30]

Though the *Junta Superior* had responsibility for the entire state, most activities focused upon the capital of Mérida and the henequen port of Progreso. The capital's team consisted of several ward leaders (*vocals*)—usually eight—with responsibilities for different sections of the city. Each representative managed all of the *Junta*'s activities in the sections, responded to cases of infectious diseases, inspected prostitutes, and conducted basic sanitary inspections. The small facility in Progreso was expanded in 1903 to include three different isolation rooms, each with capacity for four persons.[31]

The Hospital O'Horán Complex

Yucatec elites viewed the construction of a new Hospital O'Horán as another sign of the "modernization" that signaled Yucatán's position among progressive societies. The new hospital, the second major biomedical institution of the era, reflected the power and interests of the region's political elite. Olegario Molina Solís, elected governor in 1902, convened a group of people to consider a new hospital four days after taking office. His brother, Augusto, Director of the older Hospital O'Horán, had convinced him that the downtown site in a colonial building had long since proven inadequate. Leading citizens were "convinced" of the worthiness of donating to the hospital, which was to be located on vacant land to the west of the city. Leandro L. Ayala donated 250,000 pesos to catalyze the project. Salvador Echegaray, one of the Porfiriato's favorite engineers, planned the hospital based upon a facility in Milan, Italy. An asylum for the mentally ill—named the Asilo Ayala in honor of its chief benefactor—was built concurrently with the hospital.

The new Hospital O'Horán dwarfed the earlier site in scale and function. The hospital boasted 400 beds, divided among some 40 different wings that allowed for the separation of patients by sex and by types of disease. Each wing was separate from the others and raised several feet above the ground to allow the free circulation of "air so as to avoid the influences of miasmas and to permit perfect ventilation."[32] The hospital included administrative, dining, pharmacy, laboratory, and other buildings. A Department of Disinfection evidenced the increased awareness of the importance of sanitary conditions. Surgical wings were located on both the northern and southern sides of the property. The buildings totaled 46,000 square meters in a vast complex about two kilometers from the city center. Trolleys connected the new facilities to the town center.[33]

The Hospital O'Horán adhered to the model of the modern hospital established by the earlier reorganization of Johns Hopkins University, a system that linked a hospital, medical school, clinics and laboratories. Dr. Augusto Molina Solís invited the Danish physician Harald Seidelin to develop the laboratory facilities of the new hospital. Seidelin, trained at the University of Copenhagen in laboratory science, had established a practice in Mexico City in 1905 after being titled by the *Escuela Nacional de Medicina*. Dr. Ramón Alberto Pacheco recommended him to the Molina Solís brothers as they planned for the hospital's opening. Seidelin accepted a position in bacteriology and pathological anatomy, beginning his duties in August 1906. He brought various laboratory techniques to Yucatán, including the Wassermann test for syphilis and the Widal reaction for typhoid fever. Physicians associated with the School of Medicine and Hospital O'Horán used the hospital's clinics and laboratories to experiment with new medical procedures.[34] For example, Rafael Colomé utilized urine samples as a technique to diagnose patients with hysteria.[35]

Seidelin proudly announced the creation of a "museum of pathological anatomy" associated with the hospital. There he and his associates could utilize the dead for teaching purposes and the investigation of disease.[36] (Morbid anatomy was a key to nineteenth-century medical training and knowledge creation.) Seidelin helped to train various physicians before his 1910 departure for England, where he assumed a position at the Liverpool University of Tropical Medicine. Diego Hernández Fajardo and Abelardo Lara Negrón took over his position as chair of bacteriology. Hernández Fajardo later became director of laboratories at the Hospital O'Horán.[37]

The hospital adhered to more traditional principles in its fee schedule. Hospitals operated by the church or municipalities had long considered their mission to be of charitable service to the poor and disadvantaged of the community, offering their services for free. Hospital O'Horán operated as a "free" public institution. Recommendations for admissions were made by physicians or political officials, most frequently a member of a municipal council. Residents of Mérida appear to have dominated use of the facility, with limited numbers of visits by people from the henequen zone. In time, a small number of admission slots were opened on a payment basis, the onset of capitalized medical practices that generated considerable controversy in the 1930s.

Yucatán's woefully inadequate support for mentally ill residents was addressed by the Asilo Ayala. The new facility reflected "modern" notions of mental illness in which country-like conditions were thought to be better for "demented" individuals than dark, closed-in buildings. The Asilo Ayala thus had two dimensions, an agrarian colony and an asylum with two wings, one for men and women, each with 32 beds, and "in buildings [where] you could enjoy books and various manual activities."[38] The agrarian colony used sports hygiene and various manual tasks in order to avoid the "melancholy and sadness" common to many asylums.[39] During its first years of operation, alcoholism, then considered a mental illness, was the largest reason for admission. By 1917, the Asilo Ayala housed between 160 and 180 people at any given time, and treated about 2,000 people annually.[40]

The School of Medicine joined the suburban medical complex in 1911. The school moved from its downtown location into a new facility across the street from the gates of O'Horán. This intensified the use of the hospital as a training facility for medical students. Students assisted members of the *Junta Superior* in their sanitary inspections and in the monitoring of prostitution. Occasionally, an advanced student might be sent to an interior village to treat outbreaks of disease. Medical students produced as well as consumed medical knowledge. Andrés Sáenz, for example, used the Hospital O'Horán as the site for human research for his medical thesis research on the treatment of tetanus; he later presented the research to the Mexican Academy of Medicine in 1910.[41]

In 1903, formal programs in nursing education began at the School of Medicine. Governor Molina Solís supported legislature that permitted a nursing career at the school, which welcomed twelve students in that year. Initially students were required to have had earlier nursing experience. Students in nursing joined their medical counterparts in gaining experience at the hospital, as well as in the treatment of disease outbreaks. Midwifery operated as a second track until the 1930s, when the two programs merged.[42]

Professional organizations empowered biomedical physicians with the capacity to influence public policy and to expand the biomedical institutional network. They served as a critical source of identity as physicians sought privileged authority to define "legitimate" medical practices. Dr. Francisco Losa y Domínguez, a physician associated with Hospital O'Horán, played an important role in the 1905 founding of the *Sociedad Médica Yucateca*, the most influential long-term medical organization in the state.[43] Many Society members held political positions, which they used to enhance public health initiatives and medical authority. Within 15 years of its founding, the *Sociedad Médica* numbered almost ninety members, perhaps half of the titled physicians in the state. SMY members would be at the forefront of every major public health initiative through the 1940s. They would play leading roles in two medical syndicates, the *Asociación Médica Mexicana* (Mexican Medical Association, 1922) and the *Asociación de Médicos y Profesionistas Conexos de Yucatán* (The Yucatec Association of Physicians and Allied Professionals, 1934). *La Revista Médica de Yucatán*, the mouthpiece of the organization, published from 1905 through the mid-1950s, revealing in its articles and advertisements the connections between members of the organization and the larger Atlantic medical community.

Professional organs published local, national, and international medical findings. *La Emulación*, publishing in the 1870s, tended to report on research by local physicians into water quality and case studies.[44] *La Crónica Médica de Yucatán* (1890s) and *La Revista Médica de Yucatán* (1905+) included more international reports. The former, for example, included information on a vaccine that Robert Koch was developing for tuberculosis and methods for artificially breaking limbs.[45] The *Boletín de Higiene*, published in the late 1890s by the *Junta Superior de Salubridad*, offered detailed information on the activities of the organization. These included summaries of their sanitary inspections, smallpox vaccination reports, and recommendations as to the improvement of public hygiene.[46] All papers include advertisements for medical supplies, many of which came from abroad.

The 1917 creation of the *Dirección General de Salubridad e Higiene* (General Directory of Health and Hygiene) signaled a significant expansion of the activities of the *Junta Superior de Sanidad.* The new department reflected an expanded status of public health within the state political administration, and additional duties for the *Junta Superior.* A new building demonstrated the reinvigoration of the *Junta.* Directors at the dedication used grandiose language: a "majestic and imposing building" with "spacious salons," and "ample departments and galleries." For one, it "seemed as if the building was illuminated by the smile of science." Quite appropriately, "most of the intellectuals" and "civilized residents" of the city attended the solemn opening of the new facility.[47]

The increased importance of laboratory science was clear in the new facility. Amplified sanitary and inspection capacities were available to the five sections of the *Junta.* The Bromatology Laboratory tested the quality of milk, alcoholic beverages, and a broad range of foodstuffs. Concern for the quality of milk led Dr. Hircano Ayuso to lament that a child's death from milk sold on the street illustrated the divide between sanitation and the negative pursuit of "private interests," a struggle that could be won only through laboratory facilities and sanitary vigilance. The anti-larval unit sought to control mosquitoes that spread either malaria or yellow fever. The Smallpox Vaccine Institute now had the laboratory capacity to produce sufficient quantities of vaccine to sustain the anti-smallpox campaign.[48]

Disease pushed the *Junta Superior* outside the confines of Mérida. Auxiliary health units had begun under the regimen of General Salvador Alvarado. A smallpox epidemic in 1915 during the military occupation led to the creation of auxiliary sanitation units that would vaccinate people in the primary towns of the interior. Sanitary delegations were established in Progreso, Motul, Izamel, Tekax, Ticul, Tixkokob, Espita, Húnucmá, Maxcanú, Tecoh, and Temax.[49] The bodies operated throughout the state in its smallpox vaccination campaign, and in response to the outbreak of diseases, but these efforts faded with the decline of the outbreak. They were revived during the 1918–19 influenza epidemic and were thereafter institutionalized in the 1920s.

The *Junta* would continue to inspect food, housing, and public facilities in Mérida, but in a far more systematic fashion. And, for the first time, it created a system of "Sanitary Delegates" who would live and operate in interior towns, where *curanderos* dominated healing practices. The sanitary delegates would be missionaries of science, seeking to convert into "tangible reality" the "natural right of progress."[50] They often headed the Auxiliary Health Units.

These new outreach activities distinguished the new *Junta Superior* from its predecessor. Most of these activities—such as dental inspections of school children—took place in Mérida,[51] but increasingly in the interior as well. A long-established delegation in Progreso was joined by delegates to at least ten other towns, most of which were located in the henequen zone. Gustavo Vega proudly asserted that the corps of Sanitary Delegates "would convert into tangible reality what had previously been irresolute theories, or even idealist utopias."[52] Indicative of the new reality came from Tekax, where José Montes de Oca reported in May 1918 that he had issued certificates of good health to thirteen residents and conducted eleven inspections of commercial establishments.[53] Dr. Emilio J. Arcila offered a mixed report for Espita in August of that year, with 105 good health certificates, but sanitary shortcomings in the public market, two barber shops, and both theaters.[54]

These new linkages constituted something of a double-edged sword for public health officials. They reflected not only the amplified institutional reach of the *Junta*, but also a reduced freedom of action, as both municipal governments and political organizations now made claims for improvement in local health conditions. Peto's Municipal President, for example, wrote the Governor in October 1922 that dozens of children were ill and that the *Junta Superior* should send a "competent physician" capable of fighting the measles and whooping cough afflicting the children. The *Junta* proposed sending José de C. Dzul to the community, but bureaucratic inertia delayed his departure. In December, the distraught local official again wrote the governor that two children had already died, and that the doctor that he had requested two months earlier had never arrived. The doctor finally left for Peto in mid-December.[55] Similar requests and complaints became commonplace as communities became accustomed to the new services.

JUNTA SUPERIOR DE SANIDAD ACTIVITIES, 1894–1930

The *Junta Superior de Sanidad* institutionalized a variety of public health activities in Yucatán. But what did it do? Identifying the range of *Junta* activities is made possible by a marvelous set of documents, the "*copiador de oficios*," which record the offices' daily outgoing messages. The *oficios* are generally annotated, not verbatim copies, but they do capture the gist of the message and permit an overview of *Junta* activities. Systematic records are available from 1891 until the middle of 1944; partial records continue for a few more years. The numbers of annual *oficios* vary widely, from 271 in the partial first year, to over 1200 for half of 1944. In general, a marked increase in the number of *oficios* begins in the mid-1920s. The data are invaluable in tracing the changing patterns of activities of the *Junta*.[56]

Table 2.1 Board of Health Activities, 1891–1944, expressed in percentages

	1891/93	*1899*	*1903*	*1908*	*1914*	*1919*	*1924*	*1929*	*1934*	*1939*	*1944*
Epidemiology	46	28	30	42	9	20	2	3		2	9
Public Sanitation		4	10	5	30	19	15	3	1	6	3
Sanitary Inspections	11	18	19	20	33	9	4	37	20	53	51
Laboratory Services		3	4	2		3	1		20	5	2
Legal medicine				1		2	7		1		
Anti-rabies		1			7	6	36	28	41	18	14
Regulation		1	2	1		3	8	5	4	4	3
Statistics	2	10	19	15	3	2	1	5		4	8
Administration	37	21	16	21	18	32	26	20	7	14	5

Sources: AGEY, Sección Junta Superior de Sanidad, Series Copiador de Oficios, Vols. 1, 2, 6, 11, 12, 16–19, 54, 81–89, 108–110, 131–136, 159–64, 187–190, 226–31.

Table 2.2 Board of Health Activities, 1891–1944, expressed in oficios sampled

	1891/93	*1899*	*1903*	*1908*	*1914*	*1919*	*1924*	*1929*	*1934*	*1939*	*1944*
Epidemiology	16	20	52	77	8	26	2	3		2	14
Public Sanitation		3	18	10	28	24	14	3	2	7	5
Sanitary Inspections	4	13	33	37	30	12	4	39	28	63	76
Laboratory Services		2	7	3		4	1		28	6	3
Legal medicine				2		3	6		1		
Anti-rabies		1			6	7	33	29	64	22	21
Regulation		1	4	2		4	7	5	6	5	4
Statistics	2	10	33	15	3	2	1	5		4	8
Administration	13	15	29	39	17	41	24	21	9	17	7

Sources: AGEY, Sección Junta Superior de Sanidad, Series Copiador de Oficios, Vols. 1, 2, 6, 11, 12, 16–19, 54, 81–89, 108–110, 131–136, 159–64, 187–190, 226–31.

Almost half of the actions of the *Junta Superior* during its first fifteen years were epidemiological in nature (see Tables 2.1 and 2.2). Most involved the effort to inoculate the populace against smallpox, but many involved the outbreak of diseases in the capital and *partidos* of the state. All cases of infectious diseases were supposed to be reported to the *Junta*. In January 1909, the *jefe político* of Maxcanú apologized to the board for failing to report the case of a Yaqui laborer at Hacienda San Bernando who contracted yellow fever, stating that a local doctor was initially unclear of the nature of the disease. When the diagnosis of yellow fever became clear, the report was filed, a rationale that the *Junta Superior* supported.[57]

In another instance, *Junta* officers in Mérida were called to the home of Mariana Manzanilla, unsure of the nature of her illness. The physicians reported to the city's *jefe político* that the house did not need to be quarantined, even though she was suffering from scarlet fever.[58] Far more often, quarantines and house disinfections were ordered to prevent the spread of communicable diseases. During the 1903 outbreak of yellow fever, for example,

Francisco Colomé reported that he oversaw 25 house disinfections, including seven because of yellow fever and eleven due to tuberculosis.[59]

Sanitation inspections constitute the most consistent activity of the Junta over time. Early in its existence the *Junta Superior* began sanitary inspections of local businesses, especially those associated with food and beverage production. Later, new residences were subjected to a series of requirements, including its size and building materials, latrines and water supply, and appropriate distance between the latter. As the yellow fever campaign developed in the first years of the century, Mérida's cisterns and latrines came under intense scrutiny. Officials mandated that all cisterns be covered to inhibit the development of mosquito larvae. Most inspections were routine, with warnings for any shortcomings, and fines if problems were not addressed within a month or so.

The case of "El Olympio" cafe and bar proved different. A March 1903 inspection revealed that the Spanish owner, José González, was selling milk without a posted license, and that it was adulterated as well. González appealed the 25-peso fine, arguing that since his shop was not dedicated to milk sales, it didn't need a license and that he had violated no federal statute. The appeal was denied, with the reminder that Yucatán's sanitary code prevailed in the state and that licenses were required for any milk sales.[60] As this case gained public notoriety, a local newspaper accused the *Junta Superior* of failing to systematically examine the city's milk vendors, leading to a wave of inspections and fines.[61] González eventually appealed the fine to the state's Supreme Court, which ruled against the Spaniard in 1908.[62]

Maintenance of vital statistics constituted an integral dimension of a modern public health system. Especially important were mortality and disease statistics. The *Junta Superior* collected the latter, and received the former from the Civil Registry of the State. Smallpox vaccinations were routinely reported to the agency, usually by the *jefe político* of rural municipalities.[63] Normalization of reporting took some time to develop, often because officials did not always inform the *Junta* of cases of infectious diseases, leading the body to call for more systematic reporting so that they could disinfect all necessary houses.[64] Nor were their own members completely compliant; Dr. Arturo Erosa received a 50 peso fine for his failure to report infectious diseases in his territory.[65]

By 1927, ten years after the reorganization of the *Junta Superior de Sanidad*, most of its functions had become institutionalized. Two agencies, the *Junta Superior* in Mérida, and the Sanitary Delegation in Progreso were in permanent operation. So too were a series of Auxiliary Health Boards operated in interior towns. The *Junta* itself consisted of a president, four board members, a secretary, a veterinarian, the Director of Public Works, and administrators in charge of four sections. In the four-year term of Governor

Torre Díaz (1926–1930), the Anti-rabies Service reportedly treated over 1,000 people, 900 dogs (fifty of which had been rabid), and used 699 rabbits to develop the anti-rabies vaccine. The Animal Vaccination Service administered 53,951 doses of smallpox vaccine, and also examined scores of cows, pigs, and other animals for infectious diseases. The Food and Hygiene Laboratory tested 6,112 samples of alcohol, milk, water, and other products, most of them no doubt from Mérida. Finally, the Disinfection Service treated the homes of 529 people who had suffered from an infectious disease, the largest number from tuberculosis (242 cases). Additionally, the Sanitary Inspection team managed four sections in Mérida; the Statistical Section supplied state and local agencies with disease, death, and other data; and the Veterinary Section inspected 97,250 animals in Mérida and Progreso.[66] State authorities worked closely in their federal counterparts in this all-important port.

Auxiliary sanitary delegations became far more important in the 1920s. Auxiliary Boards served as primary responders to the outbreak of disease and the regulation of sanitary facilities outside Mérida. For example, a team was dispatched to Tekax to deal with influenza; to Hocabá, Cuzamá, Sotuta, Chapab, Muxupip, and Tizimín for an outbreak of whooping cough; and to Progreso for a severe malaria epidemic.[67]

In the 1920s, correspondence associated with epidemiology declined dramatically, as yellow fever was eliminated from the peninsula and as smallpox vaccinations became increasingly institutionalized. The regulation of medical professions increased, as did the range of sanitary inspections. The anti-rabies campaign grew dramatically, mostly in interior towns, averaging almost a third of the correspondence of the 1920s. By this time, the anti-rabies campaign operated in many areas of the state.[68]

Physicians associated with the *Junta Superior* worked closely with the Yucatec Medical Society to limit the legal practice of medicine to those healers with appropriate credentials. All graduates of medical schools, newcomers to the state, and other healers had to pass a test given by the *Junta Superior* in order to earn a license to practice. Newcomer María Louisa Benito failed the test, but continued offering her services to the Mérida community. A warning from the *Junta Superior* failed to halt her practice, leading to a request to the governor to levy the standard 500 peso fine upon Benito.[69] The authorization of biomedical practitioners began in earnest in 1924, when the *Junta Superior* distributed circulars warning that all dentists and physicians must be licensed, or suffer prosecution to the fullest extent of the law.[70] Similar warnings were sent to municipal councils throughout the state.[71] Thus in December 1924, Mérida police officials were ordered to arrest and deliver Alvaro Fuente to the Júarez Penitentiary.[72]

The nature of sanitary inspections established earlier by the *Junta Superior* continued through this period, albeit with an increased geographical range. Fewer inspections were associated with disease, no doubt because of the decreased incidence of smallpox and yellow fever in the state. The first annual report of the newly reorganized *Junta Superior* suggested that public sentiments were coming to accept inspections in the good of the public.[73] Still, residents such as Remigio Zapata continued to be warned of the need for a health certificate—after proper drainage improvements had been made to his property—or face a fine.[74] By the 1910s, after 20 years of operation, the *Junta Superior* had settled into the Yucatec bureaucracy as one of the most complete public health systems in all Mexican states. However, Yucatán—along with the other states—would have to adjust to the new initiatives of revolutionary Mexico.

REVOLUTIONARY HEALTH AND THE RISE OF THE MEXICAN STATE

The Mexican Revolution came to Yucatán in 1915, as General Salvador Alvarado invaded the state in search of revenue and to combat the power of the *casta divina*. Though unsuccessful in dethroning the henequen elite over the long run, his creation of a reformist political party—the Socialist Party of Yucatán (*Liga Central de Resistencia del Partido Socialista del Sureste*)—changed the nature of Yucatec politics, setting the stage for years of conflict. Alvarado sought vast social changes, though his ambitious health agenda had little effect upon the activities of the *Junta Superior de Sanidad*. Gradually, however, the revolutionary government's health agenda would transform public health in the peninsula; for now, Yucatec officials continued the development of the public health system they had institutionalized in the 1890s.

Political parties created in the course of the Revolution made claims upon the *Junta Superior*. Yucatec politician Felipe Carrillo Puerto formed the Socialist Party of Yucatán during the occupation of Salvador Alvarado. When he assumed the governorship in 1922, the *Liga Central de Resistencia del Partido Socialista del Sureste* worked closely with his administration on various initiatives. Carrillo Puerto sought the mandatory hygienic inspection of all houses, a step the *Junta Superior* opposed. His administration advanced its own health objectives, closely linked to its political objectives. As the Socialist Party made inroads into municipal levels of authority, the *Liga* would inform the *Junta Superior* of local health conditions.[75] In the wake of Carrillo Puerto's January 1924 assassination, a group of *Liga* women led by Adela Villamil de Molina provided financial support for an Outpatient Clinic.[76] In 1925, the *Liga* offered the Yucatec Medical Society use of its radio network to facilitate outreach activities.[77] During a 1929 outbreak of influenza, the *Liga* asked for a physician to treat the ill in Sanahcet, whose number has passed 100.[78]

While *Junta Superior de Sanidad* activities dominated the region through the 1930s, by the end of the 1950s federal programs had supplanted state agencies. Sanitary delegates associated with the federal government played a minor role prior to the 1930s. First appointed in 1906 to work with the yellow fever campaign, they left the region in 1911, to be replaced by a member of the *Junta Superior de Sanidad*. State officials occupied the post until 1926, when Nicolás Castellanos A. assumed the position.

Federal sanitary efforts expanded in the early 1930s. Yucatec native Dr. Mario Villamil Mendoza assumed control of the Federal Sanitary Delegation in Yucatán in 1931. Over the next three years, Villamil Mendoza developed three programs based in Mérida, four centers of Rural Hygiene, and conducted various public health campaigns.[79] Each rural clinic housed a physician, nurse, sanitary agent, and assistant, who were responsible for basic medical services, including medical education, and close cooperation with various public health campaigns.[80]

The federal government maintained delegations in Celestún and Progreso as part of its Borders and Ports Service (*Servicio de Puertos y Fronteras*). The office in Celestún, the smaller, older port, maintained only a single sanitary delegate. In Progreso, however, the nine-person sanitary delegation oversaw campaigns against yellow fever and tropical disease, the bubonic plague, and venereal diseases.[81] The federal *Servicios Antilarvarios* (Anti-Larval Services) operated in Progreso and Mérida to combat mosquito-borne disease; though a shortage of federal funds hindered the purchase of oil to spread on infested ponds.[82]

The regime of Lázaro Cárdenas (1934–40) forced fundamental changes upon Yucatán's medical system, but on terms determined by local authorities. Cárdenas envisioned that rural Mexicans could be modernized as residents gained control of hundreds of *ejidos* created from private estates; he nationalized henequen estates in August 1937. Governor Humberto Canto Echeverría took advantage of a shortfall of federal funds by proposing creation of a "Great Ejido" to be managed by the *Henequeneros de Yucatán* to seemingly fulfill the revolutionary objectives of the president. State officials managed the *Henequeneros* in service of federal objectives. By design, the move preserved the financial power of the *casta divina*, though thousands of former laborers gained control over their own *ejidos*. The governor did, however, promise the creation of health care system in keeping with federal guidelines to serve the henequen *ejidos*. (Chapter 5 analyzes this process in greater detail.)

The social assistance program of the *Henequeneros de Yucatán* (ASHOY) extended public health services to regions here to fore ignored by the *Junta*

Superior de Sanidad. By 1944, the ASHOY operated 68 medical dispensaries on the *ejidos*, with 43 nurses that rotated among them, as well as a central dispensary in Mérida. Their annual budget came to almost 1.4 million pesos, employing almost 300 people, including 76 titled doctors. In that year, an estimated half of the state's population received medical treatment through their auspices.[83]

The *Hospital para Ejiditarios 20 de Noviembre* opened as part of the ASHOY in 1946. This hospital had as its antecedent a 40-bed sanitarium opened on May Day, 1940. From the start, doctors at the institution received people from the *ejidos* and conducted visits to the henequen zone, a fact that was reflected in the new structure. The Department of External Medicine of the social assistance program received between 77,000 and 129,000 visits per year during the 1940s. When it opened, the *20 de Noviembre Hospital* housed Services for Surgery, Otolaryngology, Ophthalmology, Urology, and Women's Surgery and Gynecology. In 1948, when fully operational, the *20 de Noviembre* served 3,190 workers from henequen *ejidos*.[84]

Though Yucatec officials had outmaneuvered Cárdenas in the henequen zone, the Federal Department of Public Health established several Rural Hygiene Centers in the corn zone of the state. Directors of the centers worked with state officials, especially in the anti-rabies campaign.[85] Federal agents occasionally worked with health officers of the HOY. Thus, when measles broke out at the Santo Domingo planta No. 137, Enrique Díaz Villamil (Chief of the Pharmaceutical division of the ASHOY) wrote the DSP requesting assistance. Federal Sanitary Delegate Maximiliano Vadillo Acosta dispatched medical student Alberto Pérez to attend to the problem, though not without reminding Díaz Villamil that costs for the visits were the responsibility of ASHOY.[86] Still, in 1945 SMY official Arturo Erosa Barbachano claimed that outside of the henequen zone, rural areas desperately needed hospital facilities. Erosa Barbachano urged that state and federal officials join forces to build a minimum of six 30-bed hospitals,[87] a proposal that fell upon deaf ears amid the post-World War II financial crisis.

While the *Junta Superior de Sanidad* adapted itself to revolutionary initiatives, the Hospital O'Horán and Asilo Ayala were both showing their age. In 1940, Mérida and the state had a limited number of hospital beds, with the 400-bed O'Horán supplemented only by a 20 bed facility in Valladolid. Eighty more beds were added to the HOH facility in Mérida, but the sum could not keep pace with population growth. Further, access to O'Horán became increasingly competitive as "hospitalization" for illnesses became more normative. Access had been monetized for many individuals, leading to significant disputes over the nature and purpose of the organization. Moreover, there is considerable evidence from the 1930s that individuals and political groups sought to bypass "normal" public procedures in order to obtain free service. Since political officials had earlier granted access to the facility, requests from organizations such as the *Bloque de Constituyentes* of the Socialist party, the *Camara de Trabajo*, and the *Partido Nacional Revolucionario* became increasingly common.[88] As a result, the Hospital O'Horán operated beyond capacity, serving 4,244 people in 1944[89] and 4,380 in 1948.[90]

Facilities for mental illness were equally crowded. A 1930 appeal to the governor by a senior administrator at Asilo Ayala complained that only 63 beds were available for 144 men, and that 30 of 111 women patients had to sleep on the floor.[91] The creation of the private *Beneficencia Brunet* offered services to people with the capacity to pay; still, public health facilities for the mentally ill were fundamentally inadequate. The establishment of *Instituto Neuro-Psiquátrica in* 1954, funded by the federal government, significantly expanded services[92] indicating the decline of the state government's leadership role in the development of public health facilities.

Children too faced a shortage of facilities. As early as the 1920s federal sanitary delegates had sought to raise awareness of the needs of children; the state government did not respond. Finally, the federal and state governments committed funds for a "*Hospital de Niños* (Children's Hospital), which opened in 1940. Administrators justified the new facility on larger racial grounds: "the diet of the Maya people has led to a weakening of the race and, as a result, an alarming coefficient of infant mortality. . . ."[93] Children from interior towns could now be referred to the urban hospital. Demand for access to hospital grew quickly. By 1948, an average of 149 children were treated each day at the out-patient clinic. In addition, 853 children were hospitalized, mostly for malnutrition, gastrointestinal illnesses, and vitamin deficiencies.[94]

JUNTA SUPERIOR DE SANIDAD ACTIVITIES, 1930s–44

Junta Superior public health activities had become highly bureaucratic and "normalized" by the 1930s. A typical monthly report from 1940 involved 132 persons observed by the Anti-Rabies Service, 28 facilities treated by the Disinfection Service, 472 hygiene inspections (and the issuance of 162 health certificates), a range of building plans approved by the Office of Sanitary Inspections, 40 visits by the Chemical and Pharmaceutical Section (mostly investigating the sale of drugs), and almost 3,000 animals inspected at local markets by the Veterinary Service.[95] More than two-thirds of the correspondence in 1929, 1934, 1939, and 1944 involved either sanitary inspections or the effort to control rabies. Epidemiological activities had become much less common, no doubt because both smallpox and yellow fever appear to have been vanquished from the state. Inoculations and anti-larval activities persisted, but had become routine and seldom appeared in the *oficios*.

The expansion of the biomedical system through the *Junta Superior* touched upon once routine events. During the influenza outbreak of 1918, school events or festivals had been cancelled by the *Junta Superior*. By the late 1930s, public festivals such as bull fights and parades associated with *Semana Santa* required approval from either a member of the Auxiliary Sanitary Delegate, or from the *Junta Superior* in Mérida. Thus, in January 1944 Dr. M. Vadillo Acosta informed the governor that he had granted the municipal council of Caurel permission to go forward with their planned festival. Officials of the ASHOY had certified that the town was free of epidemic disease, thus clearing the way for the fiesta. Vadillo reminded the president of the council to keep vigilant so that no illegal sales of medicine would take place and that all food and drink needed to be sold under good hygienic conditions.[96]

Sanitary inspections too had become routine. Most sanitary inspections took place in Mérida earlier in the period, but as the system of Auxiliary Health Boards developed, their geographic loci changed. Owners of facilities that dealt with the public—restaurants, theaters, or small shops—required annual inspections to earn a certificate of good sanitation.[97] Faustino Camacho, for example, sought and received a health certificate for a beauty shop in Suma.[98] In requesting certification, a firm might be forced to make certain changes before a permit might be issued, perhaps in the location of a well or in the drainage of water. Fines might well be levied if a violation by a previously certified business were noted; thus owners of the "Colonial Theater" in Mérida were told to install porcelain restroom equipment and to make sure that toilet paper was clearly visible and replaced on an appropriate schedule.[99]

Complex cases might involve several jurisdictions. Such was the case when a group of investors sought permission to construct a "Cordage and Henequen Artifacts Factory" outside Mérida. Hygiene Director Manuel Espinosa Sierra informed the governor that the basic plans met health standards, especially in concern with dust particulates. However, since the plant would operate 24 hours a day, its proposed location violated local zoning ordinances. Meetings would be necessary among investors, state health officials, and local municipal officials.[100]

Large producers might use food standards to limit competition. The "purity" of milk had long been a concern of the *Junta Superior*, with ongoing efforts to assure minimum quality and regular inspections. In 1934, the "*Sindicato de Propietarios de Establos y Expedendedores de Leche* (Syndicates of Stable Owners and Milk Merchants)" applauded the "energetic and effective campaign against milk adulterators."[101] The union asked for a list of all milk vendors, so that it could help the government in its campaign.[102] While expressing its appreciation for their support, the *Junta Superior* refused to analyze milk samples the Syndicate had sent from Progreso, insisting that only Sanitary Inspectors could collect samples. The *Junta* did promise to send an inspector, and levy a 50-peso fine if any company was found to be selling adulterated milk.[103]

Unauthorized sale of pharmaceutical medicine increasingly concerned the *Junta Superior*. A 1934 Sanitary Code forbade *tiendas* from selling drugs, leading to a spate of complaints and investigations. The *Asociación de Médicos y Profesionistas Conexos de Yucatán* applauded the measure, pledging that it would send a note to all drugstores, pharmacists, and *boticas* informing them of the new regulations.[104] State officials might initiat a case, or local representatives of an auxiliary body or municipal council might seek assurances that a drug being sold locally was legal. Thus the *Junta Superior* ruled in 1940 that the "Drops Monterrey" being sold in the capital were harmless, but it reserved the right to reverse the rule based upon further evidence.[105] In the late 1940s, Carlos Pasos Bolio served as the "State Pharmaceutical Inspector," making a monthly report of his visits to towns throughout the state.[106]

The anti-rabies campaign grew after the 1917 reorganization of the *Junta Superior*. Dogs were not required to be vaccinated, but they had to be kept within a yard and wear a collar. Owners were responsible for the behavior of the dog, and responsible for any costs associated with a bite. If a person was bitten, they would be transported to Mérida for the series of shots, along with the dog, which would be observed to see if it was rabid. The charge was two pesos a day for the observation period, normally three weeks. However, when Mateo Pech's watch dog bit a passerby, Mérida's municipal officers asked that he not be charged for keeping the animal under observation, as Pech was "notoriously poor."[107] Over the years, hundreds of dogs were impounded, though only a small percentage had the disease. While initial attention focused upon Mérida, by 1939, the anti-rabies campaign reached at least 29 communities throughout the state, a further extension of *Junta Superior* authority.

Auxiliary Health Boards became fully integrated into the *Junta Superior* over the course of the 1930s. They increasingly became first respondents to disease, and always monitored sanitary inspections before reporting to Mérida. Auxiliary Boards always included a representative from the municipal government, and at least one physician as the sanitary delegate. Securing reliable officers was not always easy; *Junta Superior* officials rejected the nomination of Otto Figueroa in Tekax, insisting that all sanitary delegates be titled physicians.[108] HOH officials such as Rubén Arcila Torro of Izamal, served on Auxiliary Health Boards.[109] Quite often medical students were sent to help with diseases in communities; the Confederation of Associated

Leagues of Workers and Peasants (*La Confederación de Ligas Gremiales de Obreros y Campesinos*) of Chankom reported cases of malaria and fevers; Efraín Acosta was sent to attend to the sick.[110]

Medical Associations and the Biomedical Corps

Yucatán's biomedical corps expanded rapidly in the early twentieth century, with most physicians concentrated in the state capital. When the *Sociedad Médica de Yucatán* was founded in 1905, physicians tended to see themselves as members of a single biomedical community. By the late 1940s however, medical specialization was deeply entrenched in the state, leading to a proliferation of agencies, many of which were members of international organizations.

Yucatec physicians established a branch of the *Asociación Médica Mexicana* in 1922. The AMM had been founded in 1919 in Mexico City as a union to represent the corporate interests of physicians. In declaring the purposes of the Yucatec branch, founders identified five concerns for the organization: medical ethics; medical science; solidarity; social and cultural activities; and political action.[111] Within a year, local membership in the AMM had risen to 94 physicians, including those active in the Schools of Medicine, Hospital O'Horán, and the *Sociedad Médica Yucateca*. Shortly after the founding of the AMM, the SYM articulated its support for the new organization's commitment to syndicalism, a pledge to unify the profession, and to expand the scientific foundation of medicine in the peninsula.[112]

A more assertive wave of medical syndicalism emerged in the early 1930s. Inspired in part by federal efforts to establish labor standards, the *Sindicato de Médicos y Profesionistas Conexos de Yucatán* (1935) sought both local and national objectives. Though some members of the SMY thought the *Conexos* too radical for local conditions, editors of the organization's publication unanimously supported the new organization. They supported efforts by the *Conexos* to "democratize" the administration of the Hospital O'Horán, arguing that it had become administratively entrenched and closed to new ideas.

The specialization of Yucatec physicians had accelerated by the opening of the *20 de Noviembre Hospital* in 1946. The hospital's newsletter identified at least eight specialized organizations. Four years later, physicians established the *Sociedad Yucateca de Pediatría*. Under the leadership of President José Lavalle Peniche, the group was admitted to the American Directory of Pediatric Societies. At the opening ceremony, three representatives of Cuban Society of Pediatrics took part in the meeting. Soon, its representatives presented at Third National Society of Pediatrics in Mexico City.[113] In 1946, Yucatec physician Pedro Magaña Erosa represented the SMY and *Sindicato de Médicos y*

Profesionistas Conexos de Yucatán at two medical conferences in the United States,[114] symbolic of increasing national and international connections.

The proliferation of specialized groups tended to sap the energies of the *Sociedad Médica de Yucatán* and the relevance *of La Revista Médica de Yucatán.* Physicians in the region were specializing, as were physicians throughout the Atlantic medical community. By 1953, at least nine organizations were active, most based in Yucatán, but many sections of national organizations were active in the state.[115] *La Revista* ceased publication in the mid-1950s and though the society continued to operate, it had lost its premier position among Yucatec physicians.

CONCLUSION

Writing in the early 1940s, Drs. José F. Díaz and Benjamín Gongora Triay proudly summarized the cooperative efforts of the federal and state governments to improve the public health of the region.[116] While evidence from the 1930s belies the harmony of state-federal relations, it is clear that an impressive institutional edifice had been constructed in Yucatán. Led by the Hospital O'Horán, the Ayala Asylum, and the Children's Hospital, the social assistance network was sustained by the government authority and the Socialist Party. The Department of Sanitation and Beneficence managed state health programs and the *Junta Superior de Sanidad.* It was joined by the Federal Sanitary Delegation that included a laboratory, anti-yellow fever and anti-tuberculosis campaigns, various inspectors, and a growing administrative structure. Rural schools begun in the 1930s, and supported by the Socialist Party, became the backbone for a system of social security that developed after the 1940s. With the creation of the Ministry of Health and Assistance in 1943, the federal apparatus to guide medical policy was firmly in place.[117]

By the late 1940s, Yucatán boasted a complex biomedical system sustained by both state and federal governments. In his 1948 address to the legislature, Governor José González Beytia asserted that a "modern hospital within a democratic administration" served as the foundation for social assistance in the region.[118] The state government supported numerous institutions, including the Hospital O'Horán, the Asilo Ayala, the Hospital del Niño, the newly organized system of "Rural Hygiene and Social Medicine," an Anti-Cancer Center, and a Center for Social Assistance. In addition, the *Junta Superior de Sanidad* supported a Hygiene Service, a Bromatological Laboratory, a Veterinary Service, a Sanitary Engineering office, a Chemical and Pharmaceutical laboratory, an anti-rabies program, a disinfection service, and the smallpox vaccination program. The Department was also involved in multiple public health campaigns, including those against malaria, tuberculosis, influenza, and gastrointestinal illnesses.[119]

For Yucatec citizens, it would be difficult—if not impossible—to escape daily contact with these biomedical institutions. Mundane activities such as dog ownership were regulated by the state. Children and adults felt the influence of public health campaigns. Sanitary and municipal inspectors had become routine aspects of urban life, especially for home or business owners. And—of course—illnesses were increasingly subject to state jurisdiction and surveillance. Whether or not residents viewed these as positive influences upon their lives, they had certainly become normal. State and federal officials had clearly succeeded in constructing a biomedical infrastructure reflective of a "modern, civilized society."

NOTES

1. Allen Wells and Gilbert M. Joseph, "Modernizing Visions, *Chilango* Blueprints, and Provincial Growing Pains; Mérida at the Turn of the Century," *Mexican Studies/Estudios Mexicanas* 8:2 (Summer 1992), 167–215; ibid., *Summer of Discontent, Seasons of Upheaval: Elite Politics and Rural Insurgency in Yucatán, 1876–1915* (Stanford: Stanford University Press, 1996), 132. For a history of the facility, see Alejandro Cervera-Andrade, "Apuntes para la historia del Hospital O'Horán de la ciudad de Mérida, Yucatán, México," *Revista Biomédica* 12:1 (Enero-Marzo 2001), 63–74. (Originally published in the *Revista de la Universidad de Yucatán* Vol. 36 (1964), 11–29.

2. Patrick Carroll uses the phrase "plexus" to describe the "ontologically dense, multifaceted, heterogeneous yet intercommunicating nature of modern science and modern government" in his study of science and state formation in Ireland. *Science, Culture, and Modern State Formation* (Berkeley, CA: University of California Press, 2006), 4.

3. Catherine Mark and José G. Rigau-Pérez, "The World's First Immunization Campaign: The Spanish Smallpox Vaccine Expedition, 1803–1813," *Bulletin of the History of Medicine* 83:1 (Spring 2009), 64–65.

4. Mark and Rigau-Pérez, "The Spanish Smallpox Vaccine Expedition," 68.

5. Heather McCrea, "White Man's Medicine: Smallpox Vaccination Campaigns in Mexico's Yucatán Peninsula" (paper presented at the Latin American Studies Association, Miami Florida, March 2000); Arturo Erosa Barbachano, *La Escuela de Medicina de Mérida, Yucatán* (Mérida: Ediciones de la Universidad Autónoma de Yucatán, 1997), 23.

6. Mark and Rigau-Pérez, 'The Spanish Smallpox Vaccine Expedition," 81.

7. *La Emulación*, January 1875; Ana María Carrillo, "Los difíciles caminos de la campaña antivariolosa en México," *Ciencias* 55–56 (July to December, 1999), 19.

8. McCrea, *Diseased Relations*, 35–43.

9. Erosa Barbachano, *La Escuela de Medicina de Mérida*, 33–35.

10. Erosa Barbachano, *La Escuela de Medicina de Mérida*, 34–35.

11. Erosa Barbachano, *La Escuela de Medicina de Mérida*, 43; Marco Antonio Palma Solís, *La educación médica en Yucatán* (Mérida: Universidad Autónoma de Yucatán, 1990), 70–76.
12. Cervera-Andrade, "Apuntes para la historia del Hospital O'Horán," 65.
13. Erosa Barbachano, *La Escuela de Medicina de Mérida,* 34.
14. Erosa Barbachano, *Vida y obra del Doctor Vado* (Mérida: Ediciones de la Universidad Autónoma de Yucatán, 1995), 292.
15. McCrea, *Diseased Relations*, 59–94.
16. *La Emulación*, January 1873.
17. *La Emulación*, January 1879.
18. *La Emulación*, February 1873, April 1874.
19. *La Emulación*, June 1874.
20. *Boletín de Higiene*, November 10, 1895.
21. *La Emulación*, January 1873. Much of this paragraph is taken from Sowell, "Race and the Authorization of Biomedicine in Yucatán, Mexico," in *Health and Medicine in the Circum-Caribbean,* 1800–1968, ed. by Juanita De Barros, Steven Palmer, and David Wright (New York: Routledge Press, 2009), 76–97.
22. *La Emulación*, November 1874, June 1875.
23. *La Emulación*, June 1875.
24. In honor of the 100th anniversary of the founding of the Escuela de Medicina, *La Revista Médica de Yucatán* published biographies of twelve "illustrated physicians." Tomo 17, No. 12, 1934, 526–31.
25. *Reglamento del Hospital General de esta capital* (Mérida: Imprenta de Manuel Aldana Rivas, 1869); *Reglamento para el gobierno interior del Hospital General San Juan de Dios de esta capital* (Mérida: Imprenta Literaria a cargo de M. Guzmán, 1869).
26. *La Revista Médica de Yucatán*, September 1924.
27. *Boletín de Higiene*, May 5, 1895.
28. McCrea, *Diseased Relations*, 54–56.
29. Junta Superior de Sanidad (JSS) to Jefe Político del partido de Ticul, Mérida, July 14, 1891, AGEY, FPE, Sec. JSS, Copiador de Oficios, Vol. 1, entry 40.
30. McCrea, *Diseased Relations*, footnote, 218–19.
31. Joaquín Patrón and Agustín Cáceres to the President of the Consejo Superior de Salubridad de México, February 5, 1903, Mérida, AGEY, FPE, Sección JSS, Serie Copiador de Oficios, Vol.11, entry 5951.
32. *La Revista Médica de Yucatán*, February 1906.
33. *La Revista Médica de Yucatán*, February 1906.
34. Efraim Gutiérrez Rivas, *Dr. Harald Seidelin: Su obra en Yucatán y algunas de sus actividades en otros lugares* (Mérida: Diaz Massa, 1951), 18–19, 22; Álvaro Vivas Arjona, editorial coordinator, *Médicos en Yucatán* (Mérida: Universidad Autónoma de Yucatán, 2010), 20.
35. *La Revista Médica de Yucatán*, November 1908.
36. *La Revista Médica de Yucatán*, February 1910.
37. Alejandro Cevera-Andrade, "Harald Seidelin. Su labor in Yucatán, México," *Revista Biomédica* 17:3 (July-September 2002), 221–23; Carrillo, "Los comienzos de

la bacteriología en México," *Elementos: Ciencia y Cultura* 42:8 (June-August 2001), accessed September 16, 2003 at http://wwww.elementos.buap.mx/num42/htm/23.htm

38. *La Revista Médica de Yucatán*, March 1906.

39. *La Revista Médica de Yucatán*, March 1906. See Cristiana Sacristán, "Para integrar a la nación. Terapéutica deportiva y artística en el Manicomio La Castañeda en un momento de reconstrucción nacional, 1920–1940," in Claudia Agostini, *Estudios de Historia Moderna y Contemporánea de México* 19 (2000): México DF: Universidad Nacional Autónoma de México, 1999), 99–123.

40. *La Higiene*, October 1918.

41. *La Revista Médica de Yucatán*, August 1910.

42. Verónica Marisol López Aguilar, Lía Esther Pérez Guerra, and Marco Antonio Sánchez Solís, *De la superstición a la ciencia: la enfermería universitaria en Yucatán* (Mérida: FEUADY, 2003), 7, 27–30.

43. *La Revista Médica de Yucatán*, March, April, 1917.

44. See, for example, *La Emulación*, March, April 1873 and February 1875.

45. *La Crónica Médica de Yucatán*, January 31, 1891.

46. *Boletín de Higiene*, May, July, October 1895.

47. *La Higiene*, May 1918.

48. *La Higiene*, May 1918.

49. *La Higiene*, May 1917.

50. *La Higiene*, May 1918.

51. *La Higiene*, August 1918.

52. *La Higiene*, May 1918. The sanitary delegates were located in Progreso, Motul, Izamel, Espita, Temax, Tekax, Ticul, Motul, Húnucmá, Maxcanú, Tixkokob, and Tecoh.

53. *La Higiene*, May 1918.

54. *La Higiene*, September 1918.

55. Municipal President of Peto to Governor, October 26, 1922, Peto; Governor to President of JSS, November 10, 1922, Mérida; President JSS to Governor, November 3, 1922, Mérida; Municipal President of Peto to Governor, December 12, 1922, Peto; Secretary General of JSS to Governor, December 18, 1922; AGEY, FPE, Sección Beneficencia y Sanidad, Serie Correspondencia (Sanidad), 1922, Caja 753 bis.

56. The *Copiador de Oficios* are contained in 226 volumes, far too many for day-to-day analysis. My research sought to analyze JSS activities beginning in 1891 and ever fifth year thereafter. In each sample year, I took notes on every tenth *oficio*. My sample years ended up being 1891–93, 1899, 1903, 1908, 1914, 1919, 1924, 1929, 1934, 1939, and 1944. The goal of examining every tenth entry was sometimes modified, sometimes because the document was illegible, other times because no *oficio* was recorded, and, in 1908, because the secretary had begun to use thin onion paper as the carbon copy of the newly typewritten notes, often resulting in only vague purple coloring. When an *oficio* was absent, I went to the next one and counted ten after that. I created nine categories of activities: Epidemiology; public sanitation; sanitary inspections; laboratory services; legal medicine; anti-rabies; regulation and licensing of physicians; statistics; and administrative activities.

57. Jefe de la JSS to Governor, January 9, 1909, Mérida, AGEY, FPE, Sección JSS, Serie Copiador de Oficios, Vol. 18, entry 483.

58. L. Guzmán and Cáceres to Manuel Palomino, January 25, 1898, AGEY, FPE, Sección JSS, Serie Copiador de Oficios, Vol. 6, entry 1124.

59. J. Patrón and Cáceres to Governor, April 2, 1903, Mérida, AGEY, FPE, Sección JSS, Serie Copiador de Oficios, Vol. 11, entry 6171.

60. Patrón and Cáceres to Juez del Disticto, March 23, 1903; ibid., to governor, March 28, 1903, Mérida, AGEY, FPE, Sección JSS, Serie Copiador de Oficios, Vol. 11, entries 6091, 6131.

61. Patrón and Alberto Correa to Governor, May 15, 1903, Mérida, AGEY, FPE, Sección JSS, Serie Copiador de Oficios, Vol. 11, entry 6371.

62. Patrón and Cáceres to Governor, April 23, 1908, Mérida, AGEY, FPE, Sección JSS, Serie Copiador de Oficios, Vol. 17, entry 283.

63. Correa to Jefe Político de Espita, December 27, 1899, Mérida, AGEY, FPE, Sección JSS, Serie Copiador de Oficios, Vol. 6, entry 1805.

64. Patrón and Cáceres to Director Registro Civil del Estado, August 1, 1899, Mérida, AGEY, FPE, Sección JSS, Serie Copiador de Oficios, Vol. 6, entry 1515.

65. Patrón and Cáceres to Arturo Erosa, April 6, 1903, Mérida, AGEY, FPE, Sección JSS, Serie Copiador de Oficios, Vol. 11, entry 6181.

66. *Informe rendido al gobernador constitucional de Yucatán c. Dr. Alvaro Torre Díaz, ante la XXIX Legislatura del Estado el 1° de Enero de 1927* (Mérida: Talleres Tipográficos del Gobierno del Estado, 1927), 98–103.

67. *Informe rendido al gobernador constitucional de Yucatán*, 98, 103.

68. Correspondence involved Hoctún, Tepakam, Progreso, Chubuena, and Telchac.

69. Gil Rojas Aguilar to Governor, July 16, 1919, Mérida, AGEY, FPE, Sección JSS, Serie Copiador de Oficios, Vol. 85, entry 798.

70. Mario Villamil, January 2, 1924, Mérida, AGEY, FPE, Sección JSS, Serie Copiador de Oficios, Vol. 108, entry 1.

71. See, for example, Rafael Ramos Abarca to Municipal President of Dzemul, January 10, 1924, Mérida, AGEY, FPE, Sección JSS, Serie Copiador de Oficios, Vol. 110, entry 468.

72. Miguel Castillo Torre to the Inspector General of the Police, December 6, 1924, Mérida, AGEY, FPE, Sección JSS, Serie Copiador de Oficios, Vol, 11, entry 468.

73. Rojas to Governor, December 27, 1918, Mérida, AGEY, FPE, Sección JSS, Serie Copiador de Oficios, Vol. 88.

74. Rojas to Remigio Zapata, January 9, 1919, Mérida, AGEY, FPE, Sección JSS, Serie Copiador de Oficios, Vol. 85, entry 631.

75. McCrea, *Diseased Relations*, 185–87.

76. *Homeopatía*, October 1939.

77. *La Revista Médica de Yucatán*, June 1925.

78. AGEY, FPE, Sec. Beneficencia, Serie JSS, 1929.

79. http://www.salud.yucatan.gob.mx/coordenfermeria.htm_accessed August 10, 2006

80. Departamento de Salubridad Pública, Directorio General, *La Oficina Central de Higiene Rural y Servicios Coordinados en los estados* (Mexico: Talleres del Imp. del Departamento de Salubridad Pública, 1937), 64; http://www.salud.yucatan.gob.mx/coordenfermeria.htm_accessed August 10, 2006.

81. Departamento de Salubridad Pública, *La Oficina Central de Higiene Rural*, 66, 69; Román Sabas Flores to Jefe DSP, Progreso, October 1, 1930, ASSHA, FSP, Seccíon Salubridad en Territorios, Puertos y Fronteras (STPF), Caja 12, Exp. 9

82. Departamento de Salubridad Pública, *Informe general*, 48–49.

83. *Informe de Señor Ernesto Novelo Torres Gobernador constitucional de Yucatán ante la XXXVI Legislatura del Estado, 1944* (Mérida: Imprenta del Estado, 1945), 116–17.

84. *Informe del Ciudadano Profesor José Gutiérrez Beytia, Gobernador Constitucional del Estado, año de 1949* (Mérida: Talleres Gráficos, Edit. Zamorá, 1949), 110.

85. See, for example, Benjamín Gongora Triay to Director del Centro de Higiene Rural, Tizimín, February 2, 1939, Mérida, AGEY, FPE, Sec. JSS, Ser. Copiador de Oficios, Vol. 187, entry 291; Luis Vazques Campos to Jefe del Centro de Higiene Rural, Ticy, March 17, 1939, Mérida, AGEY, FPE, Sec. JSS, Ser. Copiador de Oficios, Vol. 187, entry 741.

86. Maximiliano Vadillo Acosta to Governor, January 21, 1944, AGEY, FPE, Sec. JSS, Ser. Copiador de Oficios, Vol. 226, no. 99; Ibid. to Enrique Díaz Villamil, January 21, 1944, AGEY, FPE, Sec. JSS, Ser. Copiador de Oficios, Vol. 226, no. 100.

87. *La Revista Médica de Yucatán*, Tomo XXIII, No. 3 February 1945.

88. Enrique Moguel Ruz to Director of Hospital O'Horán, January 12, 1937, Mérida; Governor to Director of Hospital O'Horán, AGEY, FPE, Sección Beneficencia, Ser. Asilo Ayala, JSS, 1938, Caja 1037.

89. *Informe de Señor Ernesto Novelo Torres Gobernador*, 67.

90. *Informe del Ciudadano Professor José González Beytia . . . año de 1949*, 96.

91. Jefe Administrator to Governor, April 27, 1930, Mérida, AGE, FPE, Sección Beneficencia, Serie Asilo Ayala, Hospital O'Horán, 1930, Caja 900.

92. "Relación de obras construidas durante los sexenios 1946–52—1952–58—1958–64," AGN, FSSA, Sección Comisión Constructora, Caja 77 (Viejo) 376 (actual), No. 9.

93. *El Hospital del Niño* (Mérida: Gobierno del Estado de Yucatán, 1940), 10.

94. *Asistencia Social* 1:3 (January, February, March 1949), 45.

95. Manuel Espinosa Sierra to Governor, March 19, 1940, Mérida, AGEY, FPE, Sección JSS, Serie Copiador de Oficios, Vol. 167, entry 320.

96. M. Vadillo Acosta to the Governor, January 11, 1944, Mérida, AGEY, FPE, Sección JSS, Serie Copiador de Oficios, Vol. 226, entry 40.

97. Hernández Fajardo to the Director of the "Diario de Sureste," May 20, 1939, Mérida, AGEY, FPE, Sección JSS, Serie Copiador de Oficios, Vol. 190, entry 1043.

98. Hernández Fajardo to Faustino Camacho, September 20, 1939, Mérida, AGEY, FPE, Sección JSS, Serie Copiador de Oficios, Vol. 1667, entry 180.

99. Manuel Espinosa Sierra to Idelfonso Gómez, February 16, 1940, Mérida, AGEY, FPE, Sección JSS, Serie Copiador de Oficios, Vol. 207, entry 120.

100. Espinosa Sierra to Governor, February 14, 1940, Mérida, AGEY, FPE, Sección JSS, Serie Copiador de Oficios, Vol. 167, entry 160.

101. JSS to Governor, July 3, 1934, Mérida, AGEY, FPE, Sección JSS, Serie Copiador de Oficios, Vol. 162, entry 607.

102. Ibid.

103. JSS to Jefe Político de Progreso, July 10, 1934, Mérida, AGEY, FPE, Sección JSS, Serie Copiador de Oficios, Vol. 162, entry 632.

104. JSS to *Asociación de Médicos y Profesionistas Conexos de Yucatán*, September 27, 1934, Mérida, AGEY, FPE, Sección JSS, Serie Copiador de Oficios, Vol. 163, entry 942.

105. Espinosa Sierra to Ricardo Laviada L., January 31, 1940, Mérida, AGEY, FPE, Sección JSS, Serie Copiador de Oficios, Vol. 167, entry 120.

106. Hernández Fajardo to Carlos Pasos Bolio, July 2, 1947, Mérida, AGEY, FPE, Sección JSS, Serie Copiador de Oficios, Vol. 232, entry 1011.

107. José María Salazar A. to Jefe de Sección Antirrábico, November 21, 1934, Mérida, AGEY, FPE, Sección JSS, Serie Copiador de Oficios, Vol. 164, entry 119.

108. Salazar A. to Governor, March 5, 1934, Mérida, AGEY, FPE, Sección JSS, Serie Copiador de Oficios, Vol. 160, entry 202.

109. Hernández Fajardo to Rubén Arcila Torro, July 8, 1939, Mérida, AGEY, FPE, Sección JSS, Serie Copiador de Oficios, Vol. 189, entry 665.

110. JSS to Governor, September 20, Mérida, AGEY, FPE, Sección JSS, Serie Copiador de Oficios, Vol. 190, entries 1113, 1134.

111. AGEY, FPE, Sección Gobernación, Serie Correspondencia, peticiones, informes, renuncias, memorias, reglamentos, Caja 754, 1922; *La Revista Médica de Yucatán*, February 1933.

112. *La Revista Médica de Yucatán*, March 1924.

113. *La Revista Médica de Yucatán*, October 1950.

114. *La Revista Médica de Yucatán*, April 1949.

115. *La Revista Médica de Yucatán*, April 1953.

116. José F. Díaz and Benjamín Gongora Triay, "La higiene," in *Enciclopedia Yucatanense*, 2nd ed. (Mérida: Edición Oficial del Gobierno de Yucatán, 1977), Tomo VI, 377–421.

117. Gustavo Nigenda-López, *The Medical Profession, the State and Health Policy in Mexico,* 1917–1988 (D. Phil. London School of Economics and Political Science, 1995), 109.

118. José González Beytia, "La asistencia social y la salubridad en Yucatán, durante 1948," *Asistencia Social* No. 3 (January-February-March 1949), 42. This material was taken from *Informe del Ciudadano Profesor José Gutiérrez Beytia . . . año de 1948*. Mérida: Gobierno del Estado de Yucatán, 1949).

119. González Beytia, "La asistencia social y la salubridad," *Asistencia Social*, 42–49.

Chapter 3

Medical Communities

The biomedical project required that physicians gain exclusive authority to practice medicine, and limit the activities of other healers. Only university training and professional practices could earn the title of "*médico*," which biomedical physicians proudly claimed for themselves. Yucatec biomedical physicians labeled Maya lay healers as *curanderos*, and charlatans as those who claimed scientific knowledge, but lacked the formal education necessary for a professional title. In 1918, as public health agents sought to improve the health of citizens of the rural areas of Yucatán known as the "interior," they asserted that "the forces of *curanderismo* seek to impede the truths of science that have placed us on the natural path of progress."[1] In his history of *Medicine in Mexico,* Gordon Schendel asserted that "*curanderos* and witches (*brujos*) and their practices . . . pose a special and serious obstacle to medical progress and the improvement of the public health in much of the Republic."[2] These doctors articulated their sense of identity in oppositional terms, with *curanderos* and charlatans occupying the role of the medical "Other." Biophysicians claimed that the "truth" produced by their scientific knowledge was superior to the "traditional" knowledge that underpinned *curanderismo* and the activities of charlatans. Progress required that *curanderos* and traditionalism be vanquished and that biomedical institutions and practices become dominant and normative throughout the region.

This encounter pitted distinct medical communities against each other. The biomedical community came to exist over the course of the nineteenth century and was integral to the region's modernization agenda. *Curanderos* were located in the colonial experience, and were represented as forces of tradition constituting an obstacle to progress. The biomedical community sought to dominate the public sphere, first by opposing the "traditional" healers of the colonial medical community. Biophysicians also opposed the emergent homeopathic and spiritist communities, and railed against those they labeled as charlatans. *Médicos* utilized a variety of stratagems, inevitably sustained by their ideological linkage of biomedicine and progress. With their claims to superior knowledge and social status, biomedical physicians sought privileged status within the Mexican legal and regulatory system. This required the articulation of a shared ideology, the creation of corporate entities to advocate for their common interests, and the campaign for authorization by the state as the only "legal" healers. According to Yucatec Governor José González Beytia, these measures would "protect these [communities] from the actions of midwives, empirics and *curanderos*."[3]

Despite their success in gaining legal authorization, healers from the "colonial medical spectrum" attended to the medical needs of many Yucatec residents well into the twentieth century. The campaign for medical domination by the biomedical healing community required a long, multifaceted struggle against healers with roots in the colonial period and the medical diversification of the nineteenth century. By the end of the twentieth century, they could certainly claim success.

COLONIAL HEALING COMMUNITIES

The traditional medicine observed by anthropologists[4] in twentieth-century Yucatán is the product of Hispanic colonization. At the time of conquest in the 1540s, the indigenous residents of Yucatán spoke a common language and shared a common culture, but did not see themselves as one people.[5] Colonization created a Yucatec Maya identity in a process that Jon Schackt labels ethnogenesis—"the coming into being of a self-conscious people that has not really existed before."[6] Hispanic norms bounded and influenced this new identity and its cultural expressions, including medical practices. Spanish colonization of Yucatán did not yield absolute domination, but rather a system with social spaces in which indigenous elite retained significant strength, albeit modified by the colonial setting.[7] The *pacto colonial* enabled Spanish, clerical, and indigenous elite to maintain their respective sources of authority[8] and helped to insulate indigenous communities against intense "Hispanicization."

Unfortunately, an understanding of the medical practices of the Yucatec Maya is hindered by the nature of available sources.[9] The *Ritual de los Bacabes*, the various Chilam Balam codices, and *El libro del judío* are most frequently cited as means to understand pre-Hispanic medical practices, though they are products of the colonial period.[10] These eighteenth-century sources imagine illnesses to be caused by one of the many gods, by the actions or powers of individuals, or—most frequently—by natural causes. *H-menes*—"the ones who know"—were the most important healers. An *h-men* (*h-menes* is plural) used ritual, divination, purifications, and herbs to affect cures. *H-menes* also conducted agricultural rituals, especially involving the production of corn on *milpas*, an echo of Mayan cosmology.[11]

The role of the *h-men* in agricultural ceremonies persisted through the colonial era, even as the religious underpinnings of their rituals came under extreme pressure. Spanish Catholics insisted upon public acquiescence to the Catholic religion of the "true god," leading to the oft-noted "idols behind alters" phenomena. The *h-men* persisted as the principal healer, though with reduced socioreligious functions. Plants and animals introduced by the Spaniards increasingly appeared in the indigenous medical kit, part of a fusion that occurred between Hispanic humoral medicine and indigenous hot/cold concepts. Some scholars view the resistance to Hispanic medicine and the maintenance of medical traditions to be a "way of reaffirming their own [Maya] identity in the face . . . of their oppressors."[12] Others assert that these merged practices operated in the social spaces permitted under the *pacto colonial*, though without an overt sense of cultural resistance.[13]

Spanish colonization altered indigenous medical practices in subtle and lasting ways.[14] The primary institutions of Hispanic medicine—the *protomedicato*, medical schools, and the Inquisition—were developed in central Mexico within fifty years of conquest. The *protomedicato* had the responsibility of regulating the training of physicians, their examination and licensing, of inspecting pharmacies, and of punishing non-authorized healers. The office operated intermittently in New Spain in the early colonial period,[15] until King Philip II named Francisco Hernández as the *protomédico general* of the Indies in 1570.

In theory, all healers would have to be examined and licensed by the *protomédico*, but in practice most practitioners were unauthorized. Fully authorized healers usually attended only to the highest levels of Spanish society.[16] Although official policy relegated *curanderos* to the treatment of only natives and mestizos, the shortage of *médicos* meant that *curanderos* often treated Spaniards as well. During periods of medical emergencies, the *protomedicato* might extend short-term authorization to *curanderos* to practice medicine.[17] This tacit recognition of unauthorized *curanderos* revealed the inability of the colonial regime to create structures that could either regulate public health policies, or eliminate undesirable medical practices.[18] Once created over the course of the sixteenth century, *curanderismo* coalesced into an amalgam of indigenous and Hispanic healing activities. Taken together, these practices served as the foundations of "traditional medicine" observed in twentieth-century Yucatán.[19]

Conquest created healing communities dominated by Hispanic medical norms.[20] The process differed in peripheral regions such as Yucatán, but in all regions Spaniards defined legal boundaries and created medical institutions. *Curanderos* were not reflective of a coherent medical system, but rather a range of activities outside of Spanish medical norms. Initially, medical pluralism revealed the sharp boundaries between Hispanic and indigenous healing systems.[21] Over time, *curanderos* became part of a colonial medical spectrum reflective of a range of practices shaped by Hispanic, indigenous, and African healing practices.

TWENTIETH-CENTURY HEALERS

A wide variety of healers practiced their skills in Yucatán in the twentieth century.[22] In the rural interior, most healers practiced colonial medicine, an amalgam of Spanish and Mayan medicine. Some were more firmly rooted in Mayan patterns; all had Hispanic characteristics. By contrast, many urban healers, including biomedical doctors, homeopaths, and spiritists, utilized newly developed knowledge and approaches to healing. Other urban healers mirrored their counterparts in the interior, although without immediate ties to rural agricultural or social settings. The vast majority of the titled doctors, medical facilities, and educational institutions were located in Mérida.

*Curandero*s dominated the interior.[23] By *curanderos*, the pioneering anthropologist Robert Redfield meant a healer who treated "illness with herbal and other medical or magical means."[24] The villagers interviewed by Carnegie Institution scholars in the 1920s and 1930s referred to most healers by their Mayan names, rather than with the Spanish terms used by Mérida's biomedical physicians. Carnegie scholars identified *h-men (ah-menes)*, *dzadzac*, *pulyah*, *x-hiikab*, and *kaxbaac* healers in the countryside. The exclusively male category of *h-men* has been described as shaman-priests. *H-men* both healed and performed ceremonies associated with the *milpa* and other agricultural activities. They occupied a social status comparable to the urban *médico*.[25] *H-men* were sometimes referred to as *yerbateros* by the Spanish, though Mayan villagers referred to herbalists as *dzadzac*. Both men and women served as *yerbateros (as)*, though only women acted as midwives (*parteras*, or *x-hiikab* ["she who does massage"]). Biomedical complaints often targeted *sobadoras*, literally translated as masseuse, but most likely a term that also included *parteras*.[26] The *pulyah,* one who worked with "black magic," would be the *hechicero* of biomedical complaints.

Other healers operated in the interior. The most common were the rural inhabitants themselves practicing household (*casera*) medicine, an eclectic blend of medical practices. Biomedical healers were not permanent members of most rural communities, though they were present on occasions. The most frequent penetration of the interior by doctors came as a result of an epidemic disease such as influenza, or the smallpox vaccinators. Doctors and sanitary delegates associated with public health agencies visited more frequently after the 1920s, and some became permanent residents of important towns such as Izamal or Tizimín. Healers with a smattering of scientific knowledge that *médicos* might label charlatans also traveled from village to village.[27]

Biomedical practitioners dominated Mérida and other cities. The numbers of biomedical physicians operating in Yucatán grew rapidly over the course of the twentieth century. An estimated ninety titled physicians worked in the state in 1895.[28] A 1924 directory of physicians in Yucatán included 171 physicians, four out of five who worked in Mérida.[29] Most doctors were engaged in private practice and were not directly associated with either hospitals or public health agencies.[30] A minority of physicians were associated with hospitals, schools, and the Board of Health, although they had an enormous influence upon public policy. In Mérida, doctors worked either in the Hospital O'Horán, Ayala Asylum, or both. A 20-bed hospital in Valladolid offered free services to the poor. Biomedical doctors dominated the Board of Health and other public health agencies.[31]

Academic training and professional associations differentiated biomedical doctors from the majority of healers in the region. Most doctors had studied at the *Escuela de Medicina de Yucatán*,[32] though others were graduated from medical schools in Mexico City, France, Germany, Cuba, the United States, or elsewhere. These doctors formed various associations to promote their professional status, including the *Sociedad Médico-Farmacéutica* (1872), the *Sociedad Médica Yucateca* (1905), and the *Asociación Médica Mexicana* (1922). Doctors used newspapers such as *La Emulación* as a forum for these efforts against *curanderos*. After 1894, they added the authority of the *Junta Superior de Sanidad* in their campaign to assert the domination of biomedicine throughout the peninsula.

With increasing numbers, and the changing nature of biomedical practices, specialized practices increasingly affected Yucatec physicians. The *Sociedad Médica Yucateca* operated from 1906 onward as a representative of the entire medical corps. By 1948 however, staff at the *20 de Noviembre* Hospital belonged to this original organization, as well as the *Sociedad Yucateca de Pediatria*, the *Sociedad Médico-Quirurgical de 20 de Noviembre*, the *Circulo de Estudios Médicos*, and the *Sociedad Yucateca de Obstetricia y Ginecología*. Each group met on a regular basis, often to hear lectures associated with their occupations.[33] The *Sociedad Médica Yucateca* sponsored the region's first medical congress in 1931, and a second one in 1944.[34]

Several other types of healers practiced in Mérida. Biomedical practitioners labeled them as either *curanderos* or charlatans, often mixing the two terms in their public critiques, though the terms originated in quite distinct medical systems. *Curanderos* drew upon Mayan and Spanish traditions that had long dominated the region. Homeopathic and spiritist healers, by contrast, were relative newcomers who operated in the urban environment, but not the countryside. Homeopathic doctors had been active in Mérida since the 1850s, with several of them holding positions at the School of Medicine and the Hospital O'Horán. Spiritists arrived in Mérida in the late 1860s.[35] Non-titled healers who drew upon biomedical knowledge were described as charlatans.

BIOMEDICAL PHYSICIANS AND MEDICAL GENERATIONS

In its first century of operations (1833–1933), the Yucatec School of Medicine trained almost 350 physicians, the overwhelming majority of them men. In addition, it granted license to practice to five dozen men trained in other countries or elsewhere in Mexico. Several hundred other biomedical physicians practiced in the peninsula. Over the years, I have tracked the professional activities of some 600 physicians, recording their education, medical specializations, positions in the public health system, and membership in professional organizations, along with other information. This analysis suggests five "medical generations" among physicians, dated largely from the beginning of their professional careers and their subsequent pattern of public activities. The "founding" generation (1820–1860) was followed by a "professionalizing" generation (1860–1890), an "institutionalizing" generation (1890–1920), the "revolutionary" generation (1920–1940), and a "specialist" generation (post-1940). These generations, though perhaps somewhat arbitrarily categorized, enable me to paint a broad-brush image of the place of Yucatec physicians in different eras.

Professional associations constitute an important dimension of my understanding of medical generations. Yucatec relationships with the Atlantic biomedical community are especially clear in their corporate expressions. The 1871 establishment of "The Medical-Pharmaceutical Society" signaled the aspirations of the "professionalizing generation" of the health community.[36] Long-term institutional authority came with the 1894 establishment of "The General Board of Health," an antecedent of the contemporary *Servicios de Salud de Yucatán*,[37] and the 1906 construction of the Hospital O'Horán. These highpoints of the "Institutionalizing Generation" were complemented by the 1905 establishment of *Sociedad Médica de Yucatán*. Its newspaper, *La Revista Médica de Yucatán*, is a critical source of information between 1905 and its closure in 1953. Other newspapers, including several by homeopathic physicians, complement the *Yucatán Medical Review*'s coverage of the first half of the twentieth century. Members of the "Revolutionary Generation" founded two medical syndicates, the "Mexican Association of Medicine" (1922) and the *Asociación de Médicos y Professionistas Conexos de*

Yucatán (1934). This generation aggressively pursued a biomedical monopoly, leading to several campaigns against "unauthorized" healers. They were active in various programs stimulated by the federal government, notably the social assistance section of the *Henequeneros de Yucatán*, a body designed to bring health care to rural residents associated with newly expropriated henequen estates. In the 1940s and 1950s, the "Specialist Generation" founded half a dozen organizations dedicated to obstetrics, pediatrics, gastroenterology, and other medical specializations, most visibly in association with the Henequeneros' *20 de Noviembre* Hospital.

The corps of biomedical physicians changed character and size over time. The 1833 founding of the School of Medicine provided the state with a medical training facility, one that graduated almost 350 physicians in the next 100 years. It also accepted the transfer of 61 other physicians into the peninsular. During the 100th anniversary commemoration of the school's founding, *La Revista Médica de Yucatán* published a list of the graduates and transfers associated with the school, totaling 409 people.

This list evidences a steady pattern of growth, influenced by non-Yucatec physicians in the earlier years, but overwhelmingly local over time. Other physicians worked in the region, though we have systematic snapshots of the medical corps from only two years, 1924 and 1932. The 1924 directory of physicians in Yucatán includes the places of residence for 171 physicians, four out of five who worked in Mérida.[38] The information from eight years later is more revealing. A list of 287 medical professionals titled by the *Junta Superior de Sanidad* includes 211 physicians, 44 pharmacists, 10 oral surgeons, and 21 midwives. Of the 199 physicians with known residences, 68 percent lived in the capital, 23 percent lived in the interior, and 9 percent resided in other areas of Mexico or abroad. Other medical professions were more profoundly skewed toward the capital, with all of the oral surgeons and 90 percent of both pharmacists and licensed midwives located in Mérida.[39]

The Founding Generation

The School of Medicine looms large in the careers of the Founding Generation (1820–1860), as do labors against epidemic disease. "Heroic" accounts of Yucatec medicine in Yucatán often begin with the efforts of Tomás

Table 3.1 Medical Generations

	State	*Transfer*	*Total*
Founding	73 (71%)	39 (29%)	103
Professionalizing	73 (84%)	14 (16%)	87
Institutionalizing	127 (95%)	6 (6%)	135
Revolutionary	75 (87%)	11 (13%)	86

Antonio O'Horán y Argüello and Ignacio Vado Lugo to found the School of Medicine amid the 1833 outbreak of cholera. Both O'Horán and Vado Lugo had received their medical education abroad, in Guatemala and Paris respectfully, typical of almost one-third of the physicians of this generation. Vado Lugo led the Medical School's faculty for almost twenty years, teaching in a curriculum based upon the traditional system of prima and visperas chairs. Medical knowledge was in a transitional era, witnessed by a miasmatic interpretation of cholera, but by a willingness to turn to homeopathic beliefs as well. The Cuban healer Salvador Riera migrated to Yucatán during the second cholera epidemic, introducing homeopathic medicine to the state, an approach to healing that slowly gained strength in sectors of the medical community. In this era of ideological change, Heather McCrea emphasizes that the second cholera epidemic helped to undermine miasmatic understandings, just as John Snow established the relationship between water and the spread of the disease in 1854.[40] Snow's findings are often cited as the beginning of epidimeological sciences, which would gain great assistance from the germ theory developed in the 1870s.

Founding generation physicians labored in a weakly developed public health system. While the state and federal governments continued their joint program against small pox, a shortage of vaccine, limited resources, a lack of centralized planning, and tension-filled state-federal relations marred the effort. Struggles to combat cholera were limited to isolation and moves to control burial patterns—and a presumed spread of disease. Mérida's General Hospital occupied a seventeenth-century building that suffered from a lack of resources and political support. The establishment of the school of medicine, however, produced a range of physicians that would signal the emergence of a biomedical system.

The Professionalizing Generation

Members of the Professionalizing Generation (1860–90) sought a more systematic institutional framework for medicine within the School of Medicine, the General Hospital, and the *Sociedad Médico-Farmacéutica.* The Medical-Pharmaceutical Society operated for just over ten years after its 1871 establishment, seeking to unify "scientific" physicians in Yucatán's first professional association. The body published *La Emulación* as its voice in support of public health objectives such as medical statistics, scientific exploration of the region's plants, and training of nurses and midwives. The Society criticized the absence of a permanent, all-encompassing public health agency, especially in the aftermath of the 1875–76 smallpox epidemic. It supported physicians at the General Hospital after its significant reorganization in 1869, which included a much closer working relationship with the School of Medicine.

The careers of Manuel Arias Durán and Waldemaro G. Cantón Cámara illustrate the key features of this generation. Both were educated at the School of Medicine. Arias Durán studied obstetrics under Vado and Santos Rubio y Palomenque. Much of his clinical labor took place at the General Hospital; in time, the obstetric wing of the hospital was named in his honor. Cantón Cámara also worked closely with the General Hospital, as part of the increasingly public face of health. He was one of the founding members of the *Sociedad Médico-Farmacéutica* and worked for the health board that fought the 1875 smallpox epidemic. This prepared Cantón Cámara for a leadership role in the *Junta Superior de Sanidad* in the 1890s and in the *Sociedad Médica-Yucateca* after 1906.

Physicians with higher social standing played prominent roles in both the founding and professionalizing generations. Augusto Molina Solís, for example, was one of ten children born to a family that had migrated from Spain to the Campeche area of Yucatán in the 1700s. Several of his brothers rose to prominence through skillful roles in the henequen boom, most notably Olegario, who served as governor of the state in the early twentieth century and briefly held a ministerial position in the Díaz administration.[41] Augusto attended medical school in Paris and occupied a range of prestigious positions, including six stints as head of the School of Medicine, and director of the old General Hospital. He played a central role of convincing his brother for the need for a new hospital in the early twentieth century.

José Ricardo Sauri y Sauri was born in Tizimín to a family with recent Castilian origins. He attended College in Alabama, and started medical school in New York. He offered his surgical skills to the Union army in the American Civil War. Sauri y Sauri finished his education in Paris, returning first to Mexico City, Tabasco, and Chiapas before assuming surgical responsibility at the General Hospital/ HOH. Like many of his generation, Sauri y Sauri joined the *Sociedad Médico-Farmacéutica*, but his wealth enabled him to make frequent trips to France. His private practice—*la Casa de Salud*—boasted Yucatán's first X-Ray machine. Unlike Molina Solís, Sauri y Sauri seemingly avoided positions in the fledgling public health system, perhaps because his political alliances often left him on the losing side, not the recommended path to leadership.

PROFESSIONALIZATION AND BIOMEDICAL AUTHORIZATION

The professionalization of Yucatán's medical corps involved a complex set of objectives. Corporate associations symbolized the professionalization of Yucatán's medical corps.[42] Biomedical practitioners sought a medical monopoly, the spread of a particular pattern of medical knowledge, the creation of medical infrastructure, personal social mobility, and the advancement of their sense of progress. Attacks on *curanderos*, spiritists, and homeopathic healers strengthened the biomedical community, forging solidarities bounded by a common medical ideology.

The *Sociedad Médico-Farmacéutica* represented an initial effort to unite members of Mérida's medical community. It numbered fewer than two dozen members and survived for about ten years. The Medical-Pharmaceutical Society founded the newspaper *La Emulación* as its mouthpiece and vehicle in support of four professional goals, including the "fight against *charlatanismo* and *empirismo* whose pernicious influences are the origin of so many negative consequences that afflict humanity."[43]

The *Sociedad Médico-Farmacéutica* advocated the development of public health systems in Yucatán, at least partially to combat *curanderismo*. Its leaders noted that during periods of epidemic disease, such as during the cholera outbreak of the 1830s, political officials would authorize the creation of a Board of Health. After the crisis passed, the Board would be disbanded. Physicians associated with the Society argued for a permanent Board with an amplified jurisdiction. The Society suggested that the lack of medical statistics hampered public health initiatives. For example, doctors had a very poor understanding of the cause of most deaths in the region, primarily because *curanderos*, *yerbateros*, or charlatans treated most people. The Society therefore proposed that municipal leaders should require a medical certificate from a titled physician stating the cause of death before a person could be buried in municipal plots. This strategy, it was reasoned, would both improve the quality of medical statistics and reduce the number of noncertified doctors.[44]

Several types of healers drew the attention of the Society. "Indian" midwives so aggravated members of organization that the Society sought—unsuccessfully in the end—to create a program of obstetrics at the General Hospital to train midwives.[45] They also accused certain nurses at the hospital with "partial" knowledge of administering medicine outside of the institution, a practice the Society labeled as a form of charlatanism.[46] Pharmacists who did not seek the advice of doctors before prescribing drugs might also earn the charlatan label.[47] Political authorities were needed in the resolution of all of these cases, but, in the opinion of *La Emulación*'s editors, many political bosses "not only tolerated the illegal practice of medicine, but generally serve as accomplices to the charlatans, and even hid them" from public attention.[48]

Yerbateros posed a particularly difficult problem for biomedical physicians. Most herbalists operated in rural areas where "rustic people" favored their services, in part because *yerbateros* were members of the local community. Indeed, rural dwellers were accused of preferring to "die in their houses" than to seek out the services of "academics or professors of medicine."[49] Unfortunately, not only "rustics" sought out *yerbateros*; so too did some members of the elite in the capital city. Only concerted action by members of the medical community could remedy the situation.[50]

The Institutionalizing Generation

The creation and reformation of public health agencies dominated the Institutionalizing Generation (1890–1920). These include the establishment of the *Junta Superior de Sanidad* (1894); the 1906 construction of the Asilo Ayala and the vastly expanded Hospital O'Horán; the passage of public health code in 1891 and its reformulation in 1912; and a major reorganization of the curriculum of the School of Medicine. Scores of physicians were involved in these organizations and were members of *La Sociedad Médica Yucateca.* Many members of this generation joined other professional organizations later in their careers.

The capacity of the new public health infrastructure created around the turn of the century was revealed in campaigns against smallpox and yellow fever. Though efforts had been made to vaccinate residents of the state, not until the late 1880s was vaccination made mandatory. McCrea argues that an outbreak in the late 1890s saw a redoubled effort, as is clear in the record of the *Junta Superior de Sanidad.* Communication between that body and municipal council contained scores of references to delivery of vaccine, or shortages in certain areas. Yellow fever struck the region of Dzitás in 1903, leading the *Junta* to dispatch Waldemaro Cantón to the town. *Junta* officials were well-equipped to join forces with the federal government's campaign against yellow fever that utilized the knowledge and technologies of mosquito control developed in occupied Cuba. State officials continued the program when the federal health officials withdrew from the region amid the Revolution in 1911.

Alonso Escalante Ávila and Alberto Guerrero Berrón offer complementary images of the institutionalizing generation. The well-born Escalante Ávila graduated from the School of Medicine in 1895 and soon thereafter spent time in Colombia working with Juan de Dios Carrasquilla on leprosy. He spent most of his career as a professor at the School of Medicine. There he played a major role in the design of the Hospital O'Horán, was quite active in the federal yellow fever campaign, and joined with José Peón Contreras to found *La Sociedad Médica Yucateca.*[51] A social conservative, Escalante Ávila worked with the paternalist *Liga de Saneamiento* and used his editorial position at *La Revista Médica de Yucatán* to advocate stricter sanitary regulations that informed the 1912 revision of the sanitary code. He died in 1917 at the age of 45.

By contrast, Alberto Guerrero Berrón lived a longer life that reflected adaptation to changing currents within the Yucatec public health environment. Trained as a surgeon by Saturnino Guzmán Cervera at the School of Medicine, Guerrero Berrón graduated in 1905 and operated within the institutional structures created by Escalante Ávila and others. Guerrero Berrón was director of the *Sociedad Médica Yucateca* in the 1930s and was connected with new organizations spawned by the Revolution, including the social assistance program of the *Henequeneros de Yucatán*. With the 1946 construction of the *Henequeneros' 20 de Noviembre*, he assumed the position of Chief of Men's Surgery.

Institutional authorization of a biomedical monopoly ranked high in this generation's objectives, especially through the *Sociedad Médica Yucateca*.[52] In 1912, Dr. Narciso Suoza Novelo identified three types of "non-professional" healers in the peninsula. First, and not surprisingly, was the "plague of . . . *curanderos*." Midwives who called themselves gynecologists and venders of patent medicine were comparable dangers. Each, Souza said, claimed that they complemented the medical profession, but he complained that these "aren't the activity of doctors."[53] Public agencies should monitor and control all healers. Souza thus urged that the Society seek "congressional protection of medical science through appropriate legislation."[54]

The Revolutionary Generation and Campaigns against Medical "Others"

Revolutionary syndicalism and the slow expansion of the Mexican state compromised the "autonomy" of Yucatán's public health officials during the "revolutionary generation" (1920–1940). It also intensified the effort to authorize biomedical practitioners. Health policy became increasingly politicized, as federal intrusions amplified Yucatec sensitivities, and as a more assertive generation of physicians encountered entrenched public health bureaucracies. While the Depression reduced economic opportunities in the early 1930s and produced multiple tensions within the biomedical community, the creation of the *Henequeneros de Yucatán* social assistance program opened employment opportunities to scores of physicians.

The politicization of health care can be symbolically linked to the revolutionary regime of Salvador Alvarado in the midst of a 1915 outbreak of smallpox. Alvarado announced an ambitious public health agenda, but did little to carry his revolutionary vision to fruition. Felipe Carrillo Puerto, his Yucatec lieutenant, assisted the revolutionary mission by the creation of the Socialist Party of the Southeast, an organization that supported his 1922 election as governor. The governor appointed psychiatrist Eduardo Urzaiz Rodríguez to become rector of the newly created National University of the Southeast;

Urzaiz promptly engineered the creation of School of Homeopathy within the university, in keeping with many revolutionary supporters, but not supported by nonsocialist physicians.

Like Alvarado, Carrillo Puerto's revolutionary rhetoric exceeded his public health accomplishments, but the establishment of a Yucatec chapter of the AMM signaled an initial alignment between physicians in Mérida and Mexico City. Yucatec public health officials were less accommodating to efforts of the federal *Departamento de Salubridad Pública* to subordinate local physicians and the *Junta Superior de Sanidad* to the authority of the revolutionary government in the late 1920s.

The 1918 reorganization of the *Junta Superior de Sanidad* signaled increasingly assertive actions to regulate the practice of medicine in Yucatán. All titled surgeons, dentists, pharmacists, and doctors were required to register to have their legal status confirmed. They would then have to pass an examination to verify their knowledge.[55] The *Junta* demonstrated its legal muscle when it fined Enrique Wanovichtz 500 pesos gold for repeated violations of sanitary code's stipulation that a physician be titled and authorized in order to practice medicine.[56]

Physicians throughout the country utilized revolutionary corporatism in pursuit of their common objectives. In 1919, physicians in Mexico City organized the AMM. Supported by the National Academy of Medicine, the AMM sought to found chapters throughout the nation to gain "control of the health care market" in the new revolutionary environment.[57] Yucatec physicians established a branch of the AMM in 1922 to improve the moral, intellectual, social, and material conditions of physicians, and to maintain relations with international and domestic medical societies. Founders identified five concerns for the organization: medical ethics; medical science; solidarity; social and cultural activities; and political action.[58] The AMM aggressively promoted the hegemony of biomedical physicians, mounting numerous campaigns against *curanderos*, charlatans, and spiritists.[59] Within a year, local membership had risen to 94 physicians, over half of the physicians in the state, including those active in the Schools of Medicine, Hospital O'Horán, and the *Sociedad Médica Yucateca*.

Immediately upon its founding, the AMM joined with the Yucatec Medical Society to advance their corporate interests. Early in 1922, Governor Carrillo Puerto had granted a medical title to US citizen William A. Jemmal. In the eyes of the two organizations, this appointment violated the state constitution and threatened the "fraternal solidarity" and professional honor of local physicians, a point made in appeals to the federal Department of Health, the local health board, and the state legislature. Federal authorities replied that this was a local matter in which they could not intervene, but they promised not to recognize the title at the federal level.[60]

Women were noticeably absent from the Yucatec biomedical community. Not until the 1930s did the School of Medicine graduate its first women physicians; they continued to be limited in number through most of the twentieth century. Efforts to train and organize midwives and nurses had proven of limited success. Few women gain official roles within the biomedical community outside the nursing profession.

Homeopaths, by contrast, welcomed women. In the 1920s, the homeopathic school of medicine and its companion hospital ended male domination of the medical profession. Women served on the board of directors at both institutions, and as well as on the faculty at the university. Six of the ten initial graduates of the Homeopathic Medical School were women.[61]

Homeopathic doctors proved a particular challenge to biophysicians in the campaign to limit the legal practice of medicine. Homeopathic medicine emerged in the early nineteenth century as an alternative "scientific" understanding of the causes and treatments of illness in the human body. Whereas "allopathic" medicine understood the body in terms of mechanical systems, homeopathy envisioned the actions of the "vital force" as the foundation of health and illness. Treatment adhered to the "like cures like" concept, involving small doses of herbs or drugs in place of "heroic" practices that homeopaths viewed as invasive and dangerous. Initially, these understandings of illness and treatment aroused few antagonisms within the medical community, but as allopathic approaches (biomedical) gained power and authority, homeopathic medicine came under attack as a "false" approach to healing akin to charlatanism.

Homeopathic medicine entered Mexico from Cuba in the early 1850s. Spanish physician Salvador Riera brought homeopathy to Yucatán in the midst of the cholera outbreak of 1853. Homeopaths claim Nemesio de los Santos Rubio to have been the first Yucatec practitioner. Many physicians were attracted to homeopathy, in that it brought "spirit" back into medicine. The vital force allowed "the spirit and soul to work and be united with all of the forces of the human machine; it should be considered in all healings."[62] These approaches permitted devote Catholics to reject the extreme rationalist approach of some secular physicians. It also created an affinity between some revolutionary socialists and homeopathic beliefs, in that both located healing in the broader social context.

Rafael Villamil illuminates both the compatibility and tensions between homeopathic and allopathic medicines. Born in 1834 to an elite family, Villamil earned his bachelor's in medicine in 1856. Like many of his peers, Villamil had an active political career, serving in many medical and political positions, including a brief stint as governor. While teaching at the School of Medicine, Villamil developed an affinity for homeopathic medicine, became a corresponding member of the Homeopathic Institute of the Federal District and of the Homeopathic College of Philadelphia. He helped to found several homeopathic journals in the early twentieth century, each of which drew intense opposition from allopathic physicians.[63]

Given the social power and popularity of homeopathic physicians, the *Junta Superior de Sanidad* faced a difficult task in formulating a stance toward homeopathic practitioners. In 1919, the administrative council of the homeopathic school in Mexico City asked *Junta* Director Gil Rojas Aguilar that Yucatán's state law be brought into agreement with the new federal constitution, thereby authorizing graduates of the homeopathic school in the capital to practice legally in Mérida.[64] Charged with articulating a response, Dr. Romualdo Manjarrez López acknowledged that "social harmony" demanded that recognition be seriously considered. But, he insisted, the state government should not blindly authorize all titles from outside the state. Manjarrez López assured Gil Rojas that he believed the National School of Homeopathy to be honorable; but that its ideals and principles might be misguided, a coded critique of the homeopathic method. Still, it seemed "natural" that graduates of the school should be titled in Yucatán. [65]

Manjarrez López none the less recommended the rejection of the request. The stance was justified not on the grounds of belief systems—embedded in knowledge and education—but rather on the basis of state versus federal authority. Manjarrez López reasoned that authorization needed to originate at the state level. He recommended that homeopathic physicians be required to present their credentials to the Board of Health and, like graduates from other medical schools, undergo an examination to demonstrate their medical understanding.[66] Unspoken, of course, was the fact that homeopathic knowledge and practices were not valid in the eyes of the examining committee and that they would fail the exam. Manjarrez López's jurisdictional logic thus avoided the underlying differences between the two medical beliefs, placing the legal system as the arbiter of "legitimate" medical practices.

Eduardo L. Menéndez argues that organizations spawned by the Revolution were among the strongest advocates for public health programs in Yucatán. The "scientific medical solutions" envisioned by biomedical physicians were highly compatible with their own progressive ideology.[67] Homeopaths saw themselves as partners in the revolutionary process, with many joining the *Liga Central de Resistencia*, the activist arm of the Socialist Party led by Carrillo Puerto.[68] With Carrillo Puerto about to assume the governorship, physicians established the *Sociedad Médico-Homeopática de Yucatán* in late 1921 to advance homeopathic medical practices and defend its practitioners from allopathic attacks.[69] As governor, Carrillo Puerto kept his pledge to approve the new group, as well as their plans for both a "State Homeopathic Hospital" and a "School of Homeopathic Medicine." The new school was made part of the newly established *Universidad Nacional de*

Sureste de México. Classes at the school began in September 1922 and the hospital opened a year later.[70]

Homeopaths challenged numerous norms as they sought institutional legitimacy. Yucatec homeopathic physicians favored a much stronger social consciousness, which Carrillo Puerto and the Socialist Party supported, but which put them at odds with the state's elites. Homeopathic physicians advanced the role of women in medicine, a stance that Elvia Carrillo Puerto, the governor's sister, certainly approved,[71] but which was at odds with most male physicians.

After Carrillo Puerto's assassination in 1924, new Governor Torre Diaz adhered to many of the socialist principles of his predecessor, but he lacked the power (or will) to protect homeopathic medicine. The relationship between the Homeopathic School of Medicine and the *Universidad del Sureste* was abruptly severed in 1929 as the University Council denied graduates certification as "Homeopathic Medical Surgeons." It is likely that the "mixed" genders within the professorate and student body of the homeopathy school alienated Artemio Alpizar Ruz, the newly appointed director of Yucatán's public education system. Alpizar Ruz had earlier clashed with Urzaiz Rodríguez on the issue in the 1910s, and had dismissed him as university rector in 1926.[72] An appeal board denied the right of homeopathic graduates to be titled from an allopathic school, so that Torre Diaz authorized the homeopathic school to operate as an autonomous agency and grant its own degrees.[73] The *Escuela de Medicina Homeopática* operated through 1938, when political animosity led to its closure.[74] Official favor—or lack thereof—determined whether homeopathic physicians were permitted to practice medicine legally.

Spiritists, by contrast, labored without political support and were frequently criticized by biomedical physicians. Officials of the *Junta Superior de Sanidad* informed the governor in 1922 that operators of the Spiritist Center *Luz y Unión* were akin to *hechiceros*, *brujos*, divinists, and *yerbateros* in their use of sorcery, hypnotism, and other "absurd practices." Dr. Miguel Castillo Torre and two police officers visited the center, speaking with both visitors and its director, Ignacio Góngora. Several patients reported that they had been prescribed and sold various drugs, all upon the advice of a medium. Director Góngora countered that he was hardly a charlatan, since he had been in business for over thirty years. Góngora told local officials that upon entering a trance, he sought out the protective advice of doctor Francisco García A., a spirit "on the other side" who informed him of the person's illness and what medications were required.[75] Little seemingly came of this campaign; ten years later physicians complained that spiritist "centers of barbarism" still operated with the full knowledge of public authorities. *Luz y Unión* continued to practice medicine without a license, where José I. González reportedly sold a "Balsamic Painkiller" (*Bálsamo Matadolor*) without a pharmacist's permission. *La Revista Médica de Yucatán* lamented that "what a sad role that a professional [pharmacist] might be mixed up in these affairs!"[76]

Dr. Carlos Cáseres expressed his disbelief that no efforts were being made to regulate midwifery. Most midwives, Cásares asserted, were modest, moral women who did their jobs to the best of their abilities. Some, however, practiced "the occult arts." Others worked in tandem with local pharmacists, giving injections and writing prescriptions, which should be the sole prerogative of titled professionals. Midwives allegedly looked with disdain upon programs of professionalization, claiming the title of *Profesora en Partos*.[77] (Professor of Childbirths)Worse, perhaps for Cáseres, was a recent congress of nurses and midwives in Mexico City. This gathering, he claimed, was a mix of the "logical and fantasy, the reasonable and absurd." He feared the organization would declare itself to be a revolutionary syndicate and seek self-regulation, an outcome that physicians needed to prevent.[78] According to Cásares, article 4 of the constitution gave to midwives the same professional status as physicians, but that their educational training had lagged, a problem that could be resolved by a monitored professional association.[79]

BIOMEDICAL CHALLENGES IN THE COUNTRYSIDE

While most efforts to ensure biomedical supremacy took place in Mérida, municipal authorities occasionally denounced charlatans to the *Junta Superior de Sanidad.* Such was the case in 1927 when political boss Prudencio Pech from the village of Chicxulub claimed that Genaro Loría A. was presenting himself falsely as a doctor. Pech reported that Loría "is not a titled doctor," but that he did have sufficient knowledge to practice medicine in "necessary cases" and, anyway, he only charged fifty centavos a visit. The Board of Health ordered Loría to stop practicing until he could obtain the necessary permission from the Municipal Council.[80] In a similar case, the *curandero* Eduardo Peraza refused an order to cease practicing medicine, whereupon Governor Torre Díaz ordered him arrested, and offered him the choice of a 100-peso fine or fifteen days in jail.[81]

Rural dwellers had little choice but to turn to *curanderos*, insofar as most physicians worked in Mérida. This presented a distinct problem to biomedical physicians. Dr. Manuel Gamio observed that while "civilized and intelligent people" wished to suppress *curanderos* and drive them from the countryside, he held a different opinion. The countryside did not have sufficient numbers of physicians; few wished to go to the interior, where they would make very little money. As a result, *curanderos* fulfilled a vital mission; their therapies had been tested over time and most remedies aided those who sought relief.

Gamio had confidence that as the country produced more doctors, empirics and *curanderos* would be gradually replaced in rural Mexico.[82]

Radical changes in the medical curriculum offered one route toward the transformation of the countryside. Dr. Cirpriano Domínguez Rivero, from Valladolid, thought that newly graduated physicians bound for a rural practice encountered three problems. A doctor first had to deal with the "ignorance of the pueblo," a problem stemming from the simple fact that doctors did not speak Maya; most rural inhabitants did not speak Spanish. Doctors had to rely upon a translator, who was seldom trained in medicine and therefore unable to convey appropriate meanings of symptoms. As a result, misdiagnosis or poor prescriptions were common, resulting in a lack of trust for doctors among the Maya-speaking community. Domínguez Rivero disagreed with those who claimed that widespread Spanish education was the answer. It made little sense to teach thousands of people Spanish: adding Maya to curricula of medical schools would more conveniently solve the problem.[83]

From some perspectives, the interior held "dark continent" dangers for titled physicians. Domínguez Rivero observed that many titled doctors had abandoned their science while living in the interior and taken on the ways of empiricism. (Knowledge founded in experience, not scientific study.) They had turned from science to "instincts." Similarly, nurses, physician's aids, and pharmacists who claimed to know medicine, but who in fact had only partial knowledge, damaged the science of biomedicine and contributed to the lack of faith in its benefits. These practitioners with partial knowledge were assisted by rural officials, the third major problem in the region. Officials seldom enforced the rules, took favors from charlatans, and contributed to the lack of respect for authority.[84]

What then were the needs of rural medicine from Domínguez Rivero's perspective? Dedicated programs of rural health ought to be established, with three years of Maya language study required for doctors who would staff them. Rigid enforcement of existing laws was necessary, especially to deal with charlatans. Finally, public conferences on the benefits of scientific medicine could help to combat *curanderismo*.[85] Critically, these steps required increased solidarity among biomedical physicians, a challenge given the diversification of the biomedical community.

Almost twenty years after he had first called for a campaign against *curanderos*, Narciso Suoza Novelo joined Pedro Magaña Erosa to renew the struggle in 1931. In a speech before the third annual convention of Mexican medical societies, the pair suggested a strategy to end the threat to their profession. The first step was to convince the public of the benefits of medical science, accompanied by an explanation of "the dangers that accompanied the empirical assistance of the sick." Science, rather than tradition, needed to be understood by the public. It was not enough, however, to simply explain the superiority of medical science. Medical facilities should be established in rural towns and villages. Vaccinations, propaganda leaflets, and local conferences would help in the interior. In this task, local, state, and federal authorities, along with medical associations, needed to cooperate, a coordination that had been lacking to date. With these steps, a concerted campaign against non-registered charlatans could begin, demonstrating the "pseudo-scientific" nature of their practices. Pharmacists needed to be regulated much more closely, as did the drugs that they sold, especially to charlatans. Strong central authority and rigid enforcement of the law were required final aspects of the campaign.[86] As for physicians, the Yucatec Medical Society proposed a law to the legislature that only those who had a degree from National University of Southeast Mexico in Mérida would have the right to practice in the state.[87]

Medical knowledge might be used to distinguish the doctor from the charlatan, but elimination of imposters was challenging. German Pompeyo S. suggested that charlatans who worked on the boundaries of titled doctors reaped the benefits of biomedical labors. Pompeyo argued that charlatans appealed to the soul, while doctors relied upon science. Unfortunately, medical science did not always attract the public's loyalty. "The doctor has knowledge, [but] silence and austerity comes from science, which always searches for the hard truth offered as the beautiful product of investigation."[88] The implication in Pompeyo's analysis was the need to win the minds—and the hearts—of the public in order to strengthen the professional medical community. Pompeyo saw the charlatans' appeals to passions as their strongest point, making "the most delicate fibers of the soul vibrate in the masses, who are fascinated by them to the point of craziness."[89]

"*Curanderismo* is a true plague" concluded a 1933 study. Alejandro Cervera A. identified six categories of charlatans, few of which would have been active in the nineteenth century. Cevera argued that people associated with pharmacies or nurses practicing as doctors constituted an important category of charlatans. Both types, he concluded, had a little medical knowledge and often prescribed drugs without formal training. Venders and hawkers of patent medicine, spiritists, and naturalists each occupied separate categories.[90] Another physician added three more categories: titled doctors who practiced outside their specialties; doctors who had lost their titles; and students who had not yet finished their education.[91]

The definition of charlatanism had changed dramatically since the 1870s. At that time, it was limited to individuals who practiced medicine without "legitimate" medical knowledge. Occasionally, a *curandero* might also be labeled as a charlatan. The authorization campaign of the 1920s had extended to label to include anyone who practiced medicine without a title from a biomedical institution. Whereas the *curandero* existed as the early colonial other; the modern medical other was more broadly conceived. The only "true" healers were specialized, university-trained *medicos*.

REVOLUTIONARY CAREERS

Many physicians of the revolutionary generation differed in their career trajectories from earlier physicians. Ramón Carrancá Trujillo began his education at the School of Medicine in 1915, twenty years after his birth in Campeche, where his father had recently migrated from Catalan. When influenza struck Yucatán in 1919, Carrancá Trujillo was sent to Ixil to assist victims of the disease. He—and other medical students—could do little more than isolate sufferers of the epidemic, which fortunately dissipated by April. Three years later he graduated from medical school, and soon became involved in the Yucatec Medical Society. In time he became director of the Society and, in the 1930s, the head of the *Profesionistas Conexos de Yucatán*. This commitment to medical syndicalism extended to the national level. In 1942, the year of his death, he was elected Secretary General of the *Confederación de Sindicatos Médicos de la Nación*.

Felipe Santos Zetina likely graduated from the School of Medicine in 1934 or 1935, just as a major controversy surrounded the Hospital O'Horán. The Medical and Professional Association alleged in a 1935 petition to the governor that the hospital leadership had become nepotistic, corrupt, and unfaithful to its charitable purpose. Traditionally, hospital services were offered gratis, based upon the recommendation of a municipal official. Santos Zetina and other petitioners claimed that hospital officials were admitting a large of number of fee-paying patients. They were housed in well-equipped rooms and afforded good medical care; those who did not pay suffered crowded, unsanitary, and unhealthy conditions. This generational conflict split the Yucatec Medical Society, which in the end decided not to take an official stance on the complaints. In any case, Santos Zetina was soon an officer of the Medical Association, an editor of the *Revista Médica de Yucatán*, and active in the social assistance program of the *Henequeneros de Yucatán*. He joined the staff of the *20 de Noviembre* Hospital shortly after its founding in 1946.

The Specialist Generation

While earlier associations and public health institutions persisted into this era, medical specializations became increasingly common, as did linkages with agencies based outside of Mexico. The specialization of the medical corps was quite visible in the Second Peninsular Medical Conference in 1944.

Sessions were organized by medical fields, unlike the first conference eleven years earlier. José Lavalle Peniche, for example, presented on his field of pediatrics, and later helped to found the Yucatec Pediatric Society (*Sociedad Yucateca de Pediatria*) in 1948. This organization was affiliated with the American Directory of Pediatric Societies. Three delegates from the Cuban Society of Pediatrics attended a session of the body in 1950. That same year Lavalle Peniche presented a paper at the third conference of the National Society of Pediatrics in Mexico City.[92]

Many physicians used medical specializations to establish themselves. Santiago Blanco Castillo appeared on the scene in 1944. He participated in the medical conference as a representative of the surgical staff affiliated with the social assistance program of the *Henequeneros de Yucatán*. Four years later he labored at the *20 de Noviembre* Hospital, and served on the editorial board of *Asistencia Social*, the public health voice of the HOY.

International relationships permeate this generation. In 1944, Alvar Carrillo Gil, long-time head of the *Junta Superior de Sanidad*, accompanied Governor Novelo Torres to San Antonio, Texas, in order to inspect their hospitals. Both officials acknowledged the need for a dramatic modernization of the Hospital O'Horán, as neither it nor the Asilo Ayala met "modern standards."[93] Budgetary constraints delayed the improvements, which began in 1947 and then in stages to the present.[94]

Where some physicians benefited more from their privileged social rank in the nineteenth century, political connections seemingly played a greater role after the Revolution. Mario Erosa Cámara's account of his life illustrates the process. Mario's father, Vicente Erosa Leal, practiced medicine in Cansahcab, no doubt associating with Antonio Aranda, the powerful local *jefe político*. Aranda dominated the local political scene and was particularly well connected to Governor Humberto Canto Echeverría, who engineered the establishment of the HOY. Vicente was associated with the medical program of the HOY from its founding, serving as a leader of the medical section. When father Vicente died of a heart attack in 1939, his son (also named Vicente) took Mario under his wing. Vicente worked with public health official Enrique de Zavala y Díaz to gain Mario a post as a medical assistant at the HOY. Mario held this position until he graduated from medical school in 1943, when he was named as a consulting physician at the HOY office in Mérida. Within two years he had risen to Head of the Women's Service; a position transferred to the *20 de Noviembre* Hospital when it opened in 1946. His brother Vicente served first as Mérida's municipal president (1947–40), and then as a delegate to the state legislature (1950–52). As soon as Vicente gained the municipal presidency, he appointed Mario head of the city's medical services, a position he held until 1953. Unfortunately for the two brothers, *camarilla* politics had their downsides. Political machinations cost Vicente and Mario their jobs in 1954. Though Mario later returned to the hospital, his status had suffered, as had the political foundations of his medical mobility.[95]

REVOLUTIONARY INTRUSIONS

The influence of the Revolution on health care in Yucatán developed quite slowly. Not surprisingly, the creation of a federal bureaucratic medical structure, replete with legal authorization and responsibilities, added another layer in the struggle against *curanderos* and helped to further define the boundaries of charlatanism. Yucatec doctors, however, were far from pleased with all functions of the new federal entities. The revolutionary regime sought to control the production of all health care and the agents who delivered it.[96]

These federal "intrusions" sparked local opposition. In 1927, for example, local physicians petitioned the governor protesting demands from the Sanitary Delegate from the Department of Public Health that all Yucatec doctors must be registered with the Department and that they report all cases of communicable diseases in keeping with article 158 of the Federal Sanitary Code.[97] Local doctors argued that the proposal was unconstitutional, inimical to their relations with patients, and a boon to *curanderismo*. It was unconstitutional, the petition stipulated, because articles 4, 14, and 16 of the constitution gave authorization to state authorities. If the Sanitary Delegate wanted the information, he could request it from the *Junta Superior de Sanidad*, which already collected that type of data. The proposed registration would give rise to *curanderismo*, the petitioners argued, because it would damage the faith of patients in titled doctors, as well as forcing up prices. Patients would abandon titled doctors and seek out empirics, who had access to the same medicine but did not have to report to federal authorities.[98]

The syndicates spawned by the Revolution took a leading role in forging linkages between local, state, and federal concerns. The *Asociación de Médicos y Profesionistas Conexos de Yucatán*[99] complained in late 1934 that "various judges and municipal authorities" were sponsoring *charlatanismo*. According to the Sanitary Code, the registry of deaths and burials were supposed to be the responsibilities of duly authorized physicians. Local politicians, they alleged, were allowing "non-authorized" persons to register deaths and burials for their personal gain and to the detriment of the profession. The Association asked that federal authorities take appropriate steps to halt such practices.[100] Within a month, a lawyer for the Judicial Service of the Federal Department informed the governor of Yucatán of the situation, asking him to take appropriate steps to comply with the rules of the Sanitary Code.[101]

In 1934, the revolutionary regime established a body for *Servicios Médicos Ejidales* that became quite active in the henequen zone.[102] The *Asociación de Médicos y Profesionistas Conexos de Yucatán* reported the next year that a henequen *hacendado* had informed them of the activities of *curandero* Gregorio Cauich in Molas. Cauich, federal authorities were informed, "was a *curandero* dedicated to the illegal practice of medicine through witchcraft." Because Cauich was said to be in violation of federal and state Sanitary Codes, the Federal Department of Public Health was asked to take appropriate measures.[103] A flurry of correspondence brought together the Judicial Service of the federal Department, its Sanitary Delegation in the area, the governor of the State of Yucatán, the *Junta Superior de Sanidad*, and municipal officials.[104] The outcome of the case and Cauich's fate is unknown, but it represented state efforts to limit federal influence in the peninsula.

ECONOMIC CRISIS AND BIOMEDICAL SOLIDARITIES

The economic repercussions of the Depression called into question the viability of so many titled physicians. Declining economic fortunes led the editors of *La Revista Médica de Yucatán* to ask their subscribers whether or not they thought a plethora of physicians existed in the region and, if so, how it might relate to *curanderos*. Dr. Alberto Berrón Guerrero, a leader in the *Sociedad Médica Yucateca*, blamed the medical community for many of its own problems. Yes, Berrón Guerrero replied, an excess of doctors existed, but *curanderos* were not at fault. Insofar as the vast majority of physicians resided in Mérida, physicians could help themselves by moving into the interior. Rural areas lacked adequate medical care, forcing peasants to seek out *curanderos*. This, for Berrón Guerrero, was expected, since "the bulk of the population is illiterate and believes in spiritists, in *yerbateros* . . . in naturalists, in invisible doctors and in homeopaths."[105]

Surprisingly perhaps, Berrón Guerrero asserted that until rural dwellers were educated, ending *curanderismo* was "anti-humanitarian" and "anti-patriotic." Better remedies included ending the economic crisis, limiting the number of foreign physicians and graduates from the local medical school, and creating rural clinics to increase the demand for specialists. He did, however, call upon sanitary officials to end the practice of illegal medicine in Mérida, leaving more opportunities for titled physicians.[106] Dr. German Pompeyo agreed that the creation of rural clinics would deliver inexpensive care, offer physicians more jobs, and undermine the power of rural *curanderos*.[107]

Other physicians offered a distinct analysis of the relationship between doctors and *curanderos*. Carlos Caseres Pérez agreed that the propensity to settle in Mérida was highly negative. But, he insisted, *curanderos* were part of the problem. Doctors should not seek to limit the number of graduates from the School of Medicine because scientific graduates were the best weapon against *curanderos*. However, they did need to communicate better and to demonstrate the superiority of health care created by scientific knowledge.[108]

Ricardo Molina added that federal authorities had complicated the local situation by adding more and more requirements on titled physicians, while charlatans operated without oversight.[109] "Paradoxically our system tends to favor those who operate outside the law, and to weigh heavily upon those who have chosen to obey it in keeping with the ideas that come with medical knowledge and the acquisition of medical titles."[110] Local authorities also deserved some blame, in that they accepted charlatans in the absence of licensed doctors. Rural areas required, one editor wrote, the "labor of a [medical] missionary" in order to demonstrate the value of a physician, even while physicians deserved appropriate compensation.[111]

Others sought a middle ground, one that accepted the monetization of medicine through professional organizations, but which sought to maintain its human touch. Dr. V. Pardo Castello, who had arrived in Yucatán from Cuba almost twenty years earlier, acknowledged that the days of doctors as priests belonged to the past. One "must accept that medicine is a profession that one practices, not to get rich, but in order to live a comfortable and honorable life."[112] He claimed not to be a member of a professional organization, and was free to practice medicine as he saw fit. His office was a "home-like" setting that set the visitor at ease, including the large number of poorer people who sought his services.[113] Yet, as more and more doctors became associated with mutualist organizations, they were employees and subject to the expectations of the organizations. They were obligated to charge everyone between 50¢ and 2.50$ per consultation, with little regard as to the ability of the population to pay.[114]

CONFLICTS WITHIN THE BIOMEDICAL COMMUNITY

Physicians from the Yucatec Medical Society and the Mexican Medical Association dominated public health institutions for many years. In 1934, the *Asociación de Médicos y Profesionistas Conexos de Yucatán* challenged the institutional power of physicians who controlled the operations and policies at the Hospital O'Horán. Imbued with a sense of revolutionary mission—as well as the desire to shape their own professional futures, the group represented the emerging political potency of syndicates in the revolutionary state. The Association supported efforts to authorize biomedical practices, but they wished to gain power in the Yucatec public health sphere. Leading officials within the Yucatec Medical Society supported the campaign against entrenched political power, but all members did not agree with the wave of syndicalism, perhaps because it threatened their institutional power.

The *Conexos* first challenged the "medical bourgeoisie" of the state. They asserted that the Hospital O'Horán and the Asilo Ayala had become the private enterprise of a limited number of physicians, a monopoly that needed to be broken.[115] The Office of Public Beneficence managed the institutions, an office that over time became a source of political power and privilege, power that the *Conexos* thought was antirevolutionary in character. Major organizations had been created in the turn-of-the-century era of institution making, a process that forged powerful relationships between public health officials, educators, and institutions. Though both institutions had been designed to serve the public at no or limited cost, time brought more and more payments into the admission and treatment process.[116]

Younger physicians in the *Conexos* challenged that power. A petition to the governor claimed that the Hospital O'Horán and the Asilo Ayala were almost full, including large numbers of people who were paying for treatment. Many of these were referred by physicians from the School of Medicine, who profited for their services from both the School and the admitted invalid. Patients received radically distinct patterns of treatment and care. Paying *pensionistas* received attentive care, with multiple daily visits from physicians, clean sheets, and regular visits from their families. The poor, by contrast, were crowded up to twenty-five in a wing, with poor food, and only two visits a week from their loved ones. Petitioners insisted that in our "socialist system" such a situation was unjust. Both institutions should be free, with no charges for admissions, rooms, food, or treatments. The *Conexos* offered to take over administration of both the hospital and the asylum for no charge, offering a list of physicians that would volunteer their services. The new policies would sever direct linkages to the School of Medicine, though students could still gain clinical experience at the hospital.[117]

This challenge opened an organizational struggle that persisted through the 1930s. The *Conexos* demanded that the monopoly of the School of Medicine on Hospital O'Horán posts be broken. The monopoly crippled the advancement of medical knowledge and skills that might benefit the infirm, all because of political relations with the government. It described the relationship as a "governmental placenta, linked by an artificial umbilical cord to the Office of Public Beneficence."[118] Medical syndicates from Toluca seconded the challenge of the *Conexos* that they have access to the Hospital O'Horán. Doctors at the hospitals used patients to advance their private interests, not those of the general good. Syndicalism, by contrast, denied these privileges and worked for the general good.[119]

Though the power of the *Conexos* grew in tandem with the federal role in the state, the old guard remained entrenched at the Hospital.[120] A physician referred to as the "chief boss of pensionism" was forced to leave the *Junta de Beneficencia* in 1938, but he was rewarded with a position at the medical school.[121] In 1941, seven years after its foundation, the *Conexos* complained that very little had been accomplished. Equipment at the hospital was outdated, patient wings were infested with pests, and the same doctors dominated the institution. What was needed was a scientific, technical, economic, and social transformation of the facility—changes that neither the government nor the old guard physicians were willing to undertake.[122]

CONCLUSIONS

The introduction of biomedicine into the Yucatán in the nineteenth century led to a reconceptualization of what constituted a "legal" healer. Biomedical interests insisted that doctors be graduates of medical schools, titled by a public agency, and committed to corporate solidarity. After the 1850s, physicians associated with the emerging biomedical paradigm replaced the racial, religious, and social features that colonial *médicos* had used to distinguish *curanderos* from themselves, with claims of scientific knowledge and professional conduct. They created professional communities that sought and achieved the exclusive privilege of practicing medicine, as well as the legal authority and power associated with state and federal institutions. In the descriptions of *curanderos* and a new other—the charlatan—physicians revealed their sense of self, one that is visible throughout contemporary Mexico. Many "biomedical representatives" continue to "dismiss village curers as quacks or superstitious charlatans." They allege "that the people who seek such cures are fools who are easily duped by charlatans in the guise of *curanderos*."[123] Although *curanderismo* is often effective and enjoys widespread popularity, it is deemed to be a "backward" approach to healing by agents of the government and biomedical institutions. These images of *curanderos* and charlatans help to illustrate success of the biomedical project.

Biomedicine transformed the healers of the region. For most of the colonial period, *curanderos* were the only healers available to most people. The wave of early twentieth-century anthropologists conducting community studies observed that only "traditional" healers were available in most towns. Over time, biomedical physicians and public health networks came to supplement traditional methods. Elders continued to use *curanderos* and traditional healing; young people tended to seek out "modern" healers, indicative of the broader social transformation of the peninsula.[124] A team of scholars reported in the 1990s that biomedical institutions were found throughout Yucatán. Most of the fifteen towns they studied had at least one federal health program; only one lacked any federal program. The towns were all serviced by paved roads, and all but one had piped-in water. The biomedical presence had not eliminated traditional healers, who were active throughout the region. Midwives were the most common traditional healers. Biomedicine dominated the region, with traditional medicine playing an increasingly marginalized role.[125]

NOTES

1. *La Higiene*, May 1918. Italics added.

2. Gordon Schendel, *Medicine in Mexico: From Aztec Herbs to Betatrons* (Austin: University of Texas Press, 1968), 131. Italics added.

3. *Informe del Ciudadano Profesor José Gutiérrez Beytia, Gobernador Constitucional del Estado, año de 1948* (Mérida: Gobierno del Estado de Yucatán, 1949), 81.

4. The Carnegie Institution sponsored numerous scholars that produced a wealth of scholarship. These include Ralph Roys, *The Ethno-Botany of the Maya* (New Orleans: Tulane University, 1931); Redfield and Alfonso Villa Rojas, *Chan Kom: A Maya Village*, publication 448 (Washington, DC: Carnegie Institution of Washington, 1934); Redfield, *The Folk Culture of Yucatán*; and Villa Rojas, *The Maya of East Central Quintana Roo* (Washington, DC: Carnegie Institution of Washington, 1945). See also *Mérida; Su transformación: de capital colonial a naciente metropolis*, by Asael T. Hansen and Juan R. Bastarrachea M. (Mexico: Instituto Nacional de Antropología e Historia, 1984); Irwin Press, *Tradition and Adaptation: Life in a Modern Yucatán Maya Village* (Westport, CT: Greenwood Press, 1975); Menéndez, *Poder, estratificación y salud*, 343–58, passim; Marianna Appel Kunow, *Maya Medicine: Traditional Healing in Yucatán* (Albuquerque: University of New Mexico Press, 2003).

5. Restall, *The Maya World.*

6. Jon Schackt, "The Emerging Maya: A Case of Ethnogenesis," in *Maya Survivalism, Acta Mesoamericana*, Vol. 12 (Verlag: Anton Saurwein, 2001), 3–14. See also Peter Hervik, "The Mysterious Maya of National Geographic," *Journal of Latin American Anthropology* 4:1 (1999), 166–97.

7. The creative nature of colonization is often located in the *mestizaje* process. See, for example, Serge Gruzinski, *The Mestizo Mind: The Intellectual Dynamics of Colonization and Globalization*, trans. by Deke Dusinberre (New York: Routledge, 2002). The parallel process among indigenous peoples has yet to be examined systematically.

8. Pedro Bracamonte y Sosa and Gabriela Solís Robleda, *Espacios Mayas de autónomia: el pacto colonial en Yucatán* (Mérida: Universidad Autónoma de Yucatán, 1996).

9. A classic and still valuable overview is Francisco Guerra, "Maya Medicine," *Medical History* 8:1 (January 1964), 31–43.

10. Grupo Dzibil, *El libro de los médicos yerbateros de Yucatán, o, Noticias sobre yerbas y animales medicinales yucatecos* [*Sacados de los antiguos libros mayas de Chilam-Balam, calendarios y demás copios curiosas*] (México, DF: Grupo Dzibil, 1997); Ramón Arzápalo Marín, *El Ritual de los bacabes: edición facsimilar, Fuentes para el Estudio de la cultura Maya, 5* (México DF: Instituto de Investigaciones Filológicas, Centro de Estudios Mayas, Universidad Nacional Autónoma de México, 1987); Ricardo Osado and Dorothy Andrews Heath de Zapata, *El libro del judío, o, Medicina doméstico [i.e. doméstica]: descripción de los nombres de las yerbas de Yucatán y las enfermedades a que se aplican, siglo XVII [i.e.XVIII]* (Mérida: D. Andrews Heath de Zapata, 1979).

11. Juan Pio Pérez C., Hermann Berendt, and Raquel Birman Furman, *Recetarios de indios en lengua maya: índices de plantas medicinales y de enfermedades coordinados por D. Juan Pío Pérez con estractos de los recetarios, notas y añadiduras por C. Hermann Berendt, M.D., Mérida 1870* (México DF: Universidad Nacional Autónoma de México, 1996), 27, 34, 40–54.

12. *Recetarios de indios*, 9.

13. Alfonso Villa Rojas, "Terapéutica tradicional y medicina moderna entre los Maya de Yucatán," *Anales de Antropología*, Tomo 11, *Etnología y Linguistica*, Vol. XVIII (1981), 13–23.

14. The following reflects the argument in David Sowell, "Multiple Colonizations: State Formation, Public Health and the Yucatec Maya, 1891–1960," in *Crossing Colonial Historiographies: Histories of Colonial and Indigenous Medicines in Transnational Perspective*, eds. Anne Digby, Waltraud Ernst, and Projit B. Muchkarji (Cambridge UK: Cambridge Scholars Inc., 2010), 78–80.

15. John Jay TePaske, "Regulation of Medical Practitioners in the Age of Francisco Hernández," in *Searching for the Secrets of Nature: The Life and Works of Dr. Francisco Hernández*, ed. by Simon Varey, Rafael Chabrán, and Dora B. Weiner (Stanford: Stanford University Press, 2000), 55–56; Viesca Treviño, "Curanderismo in Mexico and Guatemala," 50.

16. Luz María Hernández Sáenz, *Learning to Heal: The Medical Profession in Colonial Mexico,* 1767–1831 (New York: Peter Lang, 1997), 3–5.

17. Hernández Sáenz, *Learning to Heal*, 252–55.

18. Viesca Treviño, "Curanderismo in Mexico and Guatemala," 56.

19. X. Lozoya, "La medicina tradicional en México: Balance de una década y perspectivas," in *El futuro de la medicina tradicional en la atención a la salud de los paises latinoamericanos* (Mexico DF: CIESS, 1987), 65–74, as cited in Gustavo Nigenda, "La práctica de la medicina tradicional en América Latina y el Caribe," *Salud Pública de México* 43:1 (Enero/Febrero 2001), 42.

20. For an overview of the Spanish medical system in New Spain, see Luz María Hernández and George M. Foster, "Curers and Their Cures in Colonial New Spain and Guatemala: The Spanish Component," in *Mesoamerican Healers*, ed. by Brad R. Huber and Alan R. Sandstrom (Austin: Texas University Press, 2001), 19–46.

21. María del Carmen Anzures y Bolaño, *La medicina tradicional en* México: *Proceso histórico, sincretismos y conflictos* (México DF: Universidad Nacional Autónoma de México, 1989). See also Carlos Viesca Treviño, "*Curanderismo* in Mexico and Guatemala: Its Historical Evolution from the Sixteenth to the Nineteenth Century," in *Mesoamerican Healers*, ed. by Brad R. Huber and Alan R. Sandstrom (Austin: Texas University Press, 2001), 47–65.

22. For an account of an eighteenth-century healer, Giovanni Francesco Mayoli, who came to Yucatán from Rome, see Roldán Peniche Barrera, *Yucatán: Ensayos históricos y literarios* (Mérida: Ediciones de la Universidad Autónoma de Yucatán, 2001).

23. Kunow, *Maya Medicine*, 42.

24. Redfield, *The Folk Culture of Yucatan*, 390.

25. Redfield, *The Folk Culture of Yucatán*, 308–11; Menéndez, *Poder, estratificación y salud*, 238.

26. Kunow, *Maya Medicine*, 42–43.

27. Redfield, *The Folk Culture of Yucatán*, 313.

28. J. Patrón and A. Cáceres to Jefe Político de Mérida, December 8, 1902, Mérida, AGEY, FPE, Sección JSS, Serie Copiador de Oficios, Volume11, entry 5719.

29. *La Revista Médica de Yucatán*, March 1924.

30. Menéndez, *Poder, estratificación y salud*, 237.

31. For an overview of institutionalized scientific medicine in this era, see Menéndez, *Poder, estratificación y salud*, 235–45. See also Armando Solorzano, "The Rockefeller Foundation in Revolutionary Mexico: Yellow Fever in Yucatan and Veracruz," in *Missionaries of Science: The Rockefeller Foundation and Latin America*, ed. by Marcos Cueto (Bloomington: Indiana University Press, 1994), 52–71.

32. Arturo Erosa Barbachano, *La Escuela de Medicina de Mérida, Yucatán* (Mérida: Ediciones de la Universidad Autónoma de Yucatán, 1997).

33. *Asistencia Social* 1:2 (October-November-December 1948), 48–49.

34. Congreso Médico Peninsular, *Segundo Congreso Médico Peninsular* (Mérida: Diaz Massa, 1945).

35. A brief description is found in Redfield, *The Folk Culture of Yucatán*, 317–23. See also José Juan Cervera Fernández, "Preceptos divinos y contradicciones racionales: el primer movimiento espiritista en Yucatán, 1869–1879," in Piedad Peniche Rivero and Felipe Escalante Tió, coordinators, *Los Aguafiestas: Desafíos a la hegemonía de la élite yucateca,* 1867–1910 (Mérida: AGEY, 2002), 193–238; and Kaja Finkler, "Sacred Healing and Biomedicine Compared," *Medical Anthropology Quarterly* 8:2 (1994), 178–97.

36. The organization survived from 1871 until 1880 and published *La Emulación*.

37. The General Board of Health published several newspapers, most of which lasted for only a few years. The institutional history is found at: http://www.salud.yucatan.gob.mx/content/view/29/32/ (accessed December 17, 2011).

38. *La Revista Médica de Yucatán*, March 1924.

39. Junta Superior de Sanidad to Governor, January 30, 1931, Mérida, AGEY, FPE, Sección JSS, Serie Copiador de Oficios, Volume 149, entry 89.

40. McCrea, *Diseased Relations*, 62, 65.

41. Allen Wells, "Family Elites in a Boom-and-Bust Economy: the Molinas and Peóns of Porfirian Yucatán," *Hispanic American Historical Review* 62: 2 (May 1982), 233–37.

42. Illustrative of the literature on professionalization and the "othering" of non-scientific healers are: Diana Obregón, "Building National Medicine: Leprosy and Power in Colombia, 1870–1910," *Social History of Medicine* 15:1 (April 2002), 89–108; Ricard González Leandri, "La profesión médica en Buenos Aires, 1852–1870," in *Política, médica y enfermedades. Lecturas de historia de la salud en la Argentina*, ed. by Mirta Zaida Lobato (Buenos Aires: Editorial Biblos, 1996), 21–53.

43. *La Emulación*, January 1873.

44. *La Emulación*, June 1874.

45. *La Emulación*, September 1874, January 1878.

46. *La Emulación*, May 1874.

47. *La Emulación*, May 1874.

48. *La Emulación*, January 1875.
49. *La Emulación*, November 1874.
50. *La Emulación*, May 1874.
51. *La Revista Médica de Yucatán*, March and April, 1917.
52. *La Revista Médica de Yucatán*, November 1905.
53. *La Revista Médica de Yucatán*, June 1912.
54. *La Revista Médica de Yucatán*, June 1912.
55. Gil Rojas to Governor, August 16, 1918, AGEY, FPE, Sección Beneficencia, Serie Salubridad, Sanidad, Caja 642. *La Higiene*, May 1918.
56. Gil Rojas to Enrique Wanovichtz, November 10, 1917, AGEY, FPE, Sec. JSS, Ser. Copiador de Oficios, Vol. 66, exp. 114.
57. Gustavo Nigenda-López, "The Medical Profession, the State and Health Policy in Mexico, 1917–1988" (D. Phil, London School of Economics, 1995), 305.
58. AGEY, FPE, Sección Gobernación, Serie Correspondencia, peticiones, informes, renuncias, memorias, reglamentos, Caja 754, 1922; *La Revista Médica de Yucatán*, February 1933.
59. See, for example, *La Revista Médica de Yucatán*, December 1924, June 1926, June 1931.
60. *La Revista Médica de Yucatán*, March 1922.
61. Rafael Colomé T., *La Escuela de Medicina Homeopática de Yucatán: Fundación, Actuación, y clausura* (Mérida: Talleres "Imprenta Popular," 1938), 13, 14, 18.
62. *Revista de Médicina Homeopática*, October 10, 1926.
63. *Revista de Medicina Homeopática*, August 1921.
64. The request was made on February 27 and published in *La Higiene*, May 1919.
65. *La Higiene*, May 1919.
66. *La Higiene*, May 1919.
67. Menéndez, *Poder, estratificación y salud*, 241–42; Ben Fallaw, 'The Germ of Fanaticism: Science and Anticlericalism in Postrevolutionary State Formation in Mexico, c. 1915–1940" (presented to the LASA International Congress, Toronto, Canada, October 7th, 2010).
68. Gilbert and Wells, *Revolution from Without*, 195; Colomé T., *La Escuela de Medicina Homeopática de Yucatán*, 5–7.
69. *Reglamento de la Sociedad Médico-Homeopática de Yucatán* (Mérida: Imprenta "El Porvenir," 1922), 3.
70. Colomé T., *La Escuela de Medicina Homeopática de Yucatán*, 6–7.
71. See Stephanie J. Smith, *Gender and the Mexican Revolution: Yucatán Women and the Realities of Patriarchy* (Chapel Hill: The University of North Carolina Press, 2009).
72. *Dr. Eduardo Urzaiz Rodríguez* (Mérida: Ediciones de la Universidad de Yucatán, 1977), 35.
73. Colomé T., *La Escuela de Medicina Homeopática de Yucatán*, 10–12; *Homeopatía Científica*, March 1937.
74. Colomé T., *La Escuela de Medicina Homeopática de Yucatán*, 7.

75. Gil Rojas to Governor, April 11, 1922, AGEY, FPE, Sec. Beneficencia y Sanidad, Ser. Correspondencia (Sanidad), Caja 642.

76. *La Revista Médica de Yucatán*, March 1933.

77. *La Revista Médica de Yucatán*, April 1933.

78. *La Revista Médica de Yucatán*, April 1933.

79. *La Revista Médica de Yucatán*, April 1933.

80. AGEY, FPE, Sec. Beneficiencia, Ser. JSS, May 29, June 6, 1929.

81. AGEY, FPE, Sec. Beneficiencia, Ser. JSS, September 12, 13, 1929.

82. Manuel Gamio, *Algunos consideraciones sobre la salubridad y la demografía en México. Contribución de la Secretaria de Gobernación a la Conferencia Inter-Americana de Higiene Rural* (México DF: DAPP, 1939), 27–29.

83. *Boletín Mensual del Sindicato de Médicos y Profesionistas Conexos de Yucatán*, July 1942.

84. *Boletín Mensual del Sindicato de Médicos y Profesionistas Conexos de Yucatán*, July 1942.

85. *Boletín Mensual del Sindicato de Médicos y Profesionistas Conexos de Yucatán*, July 1942.

86. *La Revista Médica de Yucatán*, June 1931. The presentation was also published as *¿Cuáles deben ser las medidas más adecuadas para proseguir la campaña contra el charlatanismo en sus diversas formas?* (Mérida: Sociedad Médica Yucateca, 1931).

87. *La Revista Médica de Yucatán*, April 1931.

88. *La Revista Médica de Yucatán*, June 1931.

89. *La Revista Médica de Yucatán*, June 1931.

90. *La Revista Médica de Yucatán*, June 1933.

91. *La Revista Médica de Yucatán*, August 1933.

92. *La Revista Médica de Yucatán*, October 1950, 224–25.

93. *La Revista Médica de Yucatán*, February 1944.

94. http://horan.yucatan.gob.mx/wp/historia/ (accessed December 17, 2011).

95. Erosa Cámara, *Epistolario de un médico*, 38–44, 56.

96. Nigenda-López, *The Medical Profession, the State and Health Policy in Mexico*, 140.

97. AGEY, FPE, Sec. Beneficencia, Ser. JSS, Caja 899, May 23, 1927. The newly formed Departmento de Salubridad issued this decree in 1923; Yucatán did not hurry to comply with this federal statute. Nigenda-López, *The Medical Profession, the State and Health Policy in Mexico*, 150–53.

98. AGEY, FPE, Sec. Beneficencia, Ser. JSS, Caja 899, May 23, 1927.

99. The Association had been founded in 1922 with direct linkages to a body in Mexico City. It coordinated actions between federal and state levels. AGEY, FPE, Sec. Gobernación, Ser. Correspondencia, Peticiones, Informes, Renuncias, Memoriales, y Reglamentos, Caja 754, January 27, 1922.

100. Archivo Histórico de la Secretaría de Salud (hereafter AHSSA), Fondo Sanidad Pública, Sección Ejercicio de la Medicina, Caja 12, Exp. 5, October 31 1934.

101. Respicio Tirado to Governor, November 22, 1934, AHSSA, Fondo Sanidad Pública, Sección Ejercicio de la Medicina, Caja 12, Exp. 5.

102. Menéndez, *Poder, estratificación y salud*, 244–46.

103. J. M. Esquivel and Luis Vega Loeza to the Jefe del Departamento del Salubridad Pública, December 30, 1934, AHSSA, Fondo Sanidad Pública, Sección Ejercicio de la Medicina, Caja 12, Exp. 5.

104. AHSSA, Fondo Sanidad Pública, Sección Ejercicio de la Medicina, Caja 12, Exp. 5, correspondence from January 11, February 23, and March 14, 1935.

105. *La Revista Médica de Yucatán*, February 1933.

106. *La Revista Médica de Yucatán*, February 1933.

107. *La Revista Médica de Yucatán*, May 1933.

108. *La Revista Médica de Yucatán*, February 1933.

109. *La Revista Médica de Yucatán*, February 1933.

110. *La Revista Médica de Yucatán*, February 1933.

111. *La Revista Médica de Yucatán*, April 1933.

112. *La Revista Médica de Yucatán*, April 1935.

113. *La Revista Médica de Yucatán*, April 1935.

114. *La Revista Médica de Yucatán*, April 1935.

115. *La Revista Médica de Yucatán*, April 1935; *Boletín Mensual del Sindicato de Medicos y Profesionistas Concexos de Yucatán*, April 1937.

116. *Boletín Mensual del Sindicato de Medicos y Profesionistas Concexos de Yucatán*, April 1937.

117. *La Revista Médica de Yucatán*, April 1935; *Boletín Mensual del Sindicato de Medicos y Profesionistas Concexos de Yucatán*, April 1937.

118. *La Revista Médica de Yucatán*, August 1935.

119. *La Revista Médica de Yucatán*, August 1935.

120. *Boletín Mensual del Sindicato de Medicos y Profesionistas Concexos de Yucatán*, August 1937.

121. *Boletín Mensual del Sindicato de Medicos y Profesionistas Concexos de Yucatán*, October 1937.

122. *Boletín Mensual del Sindicato de Medicos y Profesionistas Concexos de Yucatán*, November 1937.

123. Alan R. Sandstrom, "Mesoamerican Healers and Medical Anthropology: Summary and Concluding Remarks," in *Mesoamerican Healers*, 309, 310.

124. Ruth Gubler, "La medicina tradicional en Yucatán a través de los siglos," in Ruth Gubler, organizar and compiler, *Yucatán a través de los siglos (Memorias del 49th Congreso Internacional de Americanistas. Quito, Ecuador, 1997)* (Mérida: Universidad Autónoma de Yucatán, 2001), 229–247.

125. Yam Sosa, Quiñones Vega, and Pérez, *La medicina tradicional entre los Henequeneros y maiceros.*

Chapter 4

Disease and Public Health Campaigns

In the early twentieth century, yellow fever and Yucatán were synonymous in many people's minds. Joseph H. White, a key official in the Rockefeller Foundation, thought the peninsula to be the "seed bed" of the disease.[1] Lamentably, yellow fever was all too familiar to residents of Yucatán. It was especially common among newcomers to the peninsula, who might spark a generalized outbreak. In 1903, an influx of Chinese laborers raised fears among public health officials that they might fall ill with the disease, and that it might spread. Dr. Arturo Erosa inspected over a dozen Mérida residences in early January, finding no illnesses but very crowded living conditions. Two of the houses exceeded the twenty person per dwelling limit. Erosa informed the laborers that they needed to increase ventilation, suggesting that they open their windows during the day.[2] On May 12 Dr. Ermilo Solis reported a case of yellow fever in a house with some 80 to 100 Chinese residents, none of whom could speak Spanish. Four days later, a young Spaniard recently arrived from Cuba fell ill. By early June, a general outbreak was sweeping the city.[3] Mérida officials opened a yellow fever lazaretto for victims of the disease. In August, Waldemero G. Cantón rushed to Dzitás to assist victims of the disease in that nearby community. By the end of year, six dozen people had been sickened in Dzitás with six deaths; in Mérida 67 people died and 172 were admitted to the lazaretto.[4] An unknown number sickened and died in other communities.

Yellow fever regularly afflicted residents of Yucatán after the horrific epidemic that swept through the circum-Caribbean region in the late 1640s. The disease soon became endemic to the peninsula, joining the multiple diseases that crossed the Atlantic after 1492. The linkage of Europe, Africa, and the Americas led to the transmission of the great crowd killers—smallpox, the plague, influenza, and yellow fever—all with horrific demographic consequences among indigenous populations. Yucatán's native populations declined by at least one-half as these new diseases ravaged the population. Despite quarantines and local public health efforts, epidemic diseases ran unchecked through the region until the nineteenth century. The slow development of immunity, the introduction of smallpox vaccines, and cooperative efforts by international sanitarians finally reduced their severity, allowing for a demographic rebound beginning in the later colonial period.

Public health campaigns contributed to the declining ferocity of epidemic diseases, but did little to address the more common illnesses that plagued the region. Endemic diseases—often associated with the quality of water—had always been the leading cause of death, save during epidemic outbreaks. Early twentieth century public health officials responded to "normal" diseases less aggressively than epidemic diseases, in part because they feared diseases that might undermine export profits more than those that afflicted the general population, and in part because they lacked the social commitment to undertake more fundamental public health activities. Still, public health campaigns and sanitary efforts reduced overall mortality rates over the course of the twentieth century, leading to a significant population growth in the region.

This chapter surveys the disease environment of Yucatán within the Caribbean region. It focuses upon three periods; the colonial age of the great killers; the nineteenth-century, with initial campaigns to control smallpox; and the twentieth-century campaigns against epidemic and endemic diseases. Throughout, attention focuses upon the role of public health agents in the transformation of the disease environment, and their increased interaction with national and international actors.

THE GREAT KILLERS

Common European diseases entered the Caribbean with Columbus's second voyage. These illnesses wasted the population of the islands, but the Atlantic Ocean proved to be a remarkable barrier to the great "crowd killers" of the Old World. The epidemiology of the great killers—smallpox, the plague, measles, and influenza—help explain why the ocean inhibited their easy transfer, even as diseases such as malaria almost immediately accompanied Europeans into the Caribbean.

Though smallpox now exists in a limited number of laboratories, it was one of the most successful killers ever to afflict humanity. Smallpox is transmitted by mucous or by direct contact, and can be contracted from the dried scabies that remain in bedding or clothing. It incubates in the body for about two weeks, when the victim develops a high fever, bouts of vomiting, severe abdominal pain, and headache. At this time, the victim becomes contagious. The poxes erupt a few days later and remain for a week to ten days before drying up and falling off. About a month passes from the contraction of the disease to recovery. Smallpox tended to kill older children and younger adults more frequently. Survivors of the disease earned long-term immunity: "one either has smallpox and can transmit it, or one has not and cannot transmit it."[5]

Given that most Europeans had smallpox in their youth, immunity and the length of the Atlantic voyage hindered its transmission to the New World. The World Health Organization and a smaller number of investigators claim that smallpox appeared in the Caribbean in 1507;[6] most date its definitive arrival to late 1518. As smallpox attacked the virgin population of the Caribbean, catastrophic human deaths resulted. Within two years, the mainland suffered its first outbreak; thereafter smallpox epidemics repeatedly ravaged the region.

Measles, the second great killer, appeared in the Indies about ten years after smallpox. Like smallpox, measles was a common childhood disease in the Old World. Prior to the development of a measles vaccine in the twentieth century, about ninety percent of children contracted this highly contagious disease in the United States.[7] Measles are caused by the *rubeola* virus, which is easily transmitted from human to human, usually by mucous or by touch; it can also be airborne. Initial symptoms are flu-like in character, with lethargy, runny eyes, a high fever, and irritability. About ten days after exposure, small white spots appear in the mouth, followed two to four days later by bumps that appear on the face and migrate over the body. The infected person may pass on the disease at this stage, and will continue to be contagious almost until the rash fades a week later. Measles, like smallpox, passes through the body in less than a month and also provides immunity to the survivor.

Measles crossed the ocean in the late 1520s or early 1530s. David Noble Cook speculates that Seville was its likely origin. It possibly struck Cuba in 1529, but it clearly infected Mesoamerica in 1531, with outbreaks from northern Mexico to Guatemala.[8] Once introduced, measles periodically erupted in epidemic form before becoming endemic in population centers as a childhood disease.

The third great killer, the plague, arrived at the same time as measles. The pathogen *Yersinia pestis* causes both pneumonic and bubonic plague, but the epidemiology of the two diseases are quite different. The bubonic plague originates when the bacilli resident in rodent populations is transferred by either flea or rodent bites to humans. The disease quickly travels through the blood stream into the liver, spleen, and lungs. Lymph glands become swollen, hot, and painful, creating the buboes that make the disease readily identifiable. Blood vessels under the skin on extremities often burst, blackening the skin. Left untreated, the "black death" will come in about seven days for about half of the people infected with the bubonic version of the plague.

Pneumonic plague, by contrast, is an airborne disease and is transmitted from human to human. The sneeze of an infected person can carry the disease, which quickly settles into the lungs and almost always causes death. The coughing and sneezing fits that accompany the disease make it highly contagious.[9]

Plague was well-known in the Iberian Peninsula. A carrier of the disease would not have been allowed to board a ship. Rats, however, made the voyage with impunity and no doubt transferred the pathogen into the region.[10] Outbreaks of the plague occurred in Nicaragua in 1531, Mexico in 1545, and Brazil in 1561.[11] The pathogen remained endemic in rodent populations, thereby facilitating occasional outbreaks of the disease among humans.

Influenza, the final great killer, came to humans from pigs and ducks. Many different forms of the influenza virus exist; it mutates easily. Influenza can be a mild or severe respiratory illness, with high fevers, head and joint aches, extreme lethargy, coughs, and sometimes nausea, vomiting, and diarrhea. Most people contract the disease from droplets spread by coughing or sneezing; it can also be contracted by touch. Symptoms appear with 48 hours of infection. Influenza is highly contagious and can be transmitted before an individual realizes she or he is sick. Most people recover from influenza, though some strains of the virus are horrendous killers. The influenza pandemic of 1918–19 swept across most of the planet, killing at least 50 million people, perhaps single greatest death toll from epidemic disease in human history.[12]

It is unclear when influenza first crossed the ocean. It might have been one of the diseases that arrived with Columbus's second voyage in 1493 and spread throughout the Caribbean the next year. A disease referred to as *modorra* swept through Panama from 1514 until 1517, afflicting both native and Spaniard alike. It was clearly part of the 1530–31 pandemic.[13] Like the other great killers, once established, periodic influenza epidemics caused large numbers of deaths.

Though malaria should not be considered as a crowd killer, this debilitating disease had long been endemic to the Old World. Several types of the *plasmodium* parasite live within the *Anopheles* mosquito and causes malaria in humans. When an infested mosquito passes the parasites to a human, they migrate to the liver, where they breed during a several week incubation stage. The parasites then move into the bloodstream, where they attack and kill red blood cells, resulting in the fevers and chills that are characteristic of the disease. When an infected person is bitten by a mosquito, the mosquito serves as the vector in transmitting the disease, though it is not hurt by the parasite. Malaria kills only a small percentage of the people who suffer the disease, though the *Plasmodium falciparum* parasite is much more dangerous than others. Rather, it weakens the host, subjecting them to periodic fevers, bouts of diarrhea, and vomiting that might plague a person for years.[14]

The *Anopheles* mosquito appears to have been indigenous to the New World, but not the parasite. The many water containers on board ships that crossed the ocean provided an ideal habitat for mosquitoes, so that either they or a human could easily carry the disease into the Caribbean. Malaria crossed the Atlantic with Columbus's fourth trip in June 1502. The fleet coasted the western Caribbean from August 1502 through the following April, traveling from Honduras to Panama before seeking refuge in Jamaica to repair their damaged vessels. Once established, this debilitating disease became endemic to lowland regions such as Yucatán and no doubt increased the numbers of deaths when epidemic diseases swept through a region.[15]

YUCATEC EPIDEMICS

Yucatán's epidemiological history is distinct from that of the Mexican mainland. Several factors account for variations in outbreaks of epidemic disease in Yucatán and central Mexico. The geography of central Mexico tends toward wetter, more consistent weather patterns that sustain larger, nucleated residential patterns. The karst topography of Yucatán is coupled with less voluminous and infrequent rainfall. This led to a more dispersed residential pattern supported by shifting *milpa* agriculture. Drought and famine periodically plagued the region before contact, but efforts by the Spaniards to concentrate indigenous peoples into nucleated communities amplified loss of life during colonial epidemics and famines. During times of famine, Maya agriculturalists tended to migrate away from the scrub areas of northwest Yucatán to the high bush zones to the south and east.[16] Population shift was facilitated by the existence of unconquered zones to the south, where Maya might seek refuge from the world of the *dzul* (foreigner).[17]

Indigenous accounts suggest that widespread disease characterized Katuns 1 Ahua and 12 Ahua (1638–77). These likely include a "new" killer, yellow

Table 4.1 Yucatec Epidemics, 1519–1920

1519	Smallpox	1799	vómito de sangre
1566	epidemic	1809–10	epidemic
1575–76	epidemic	1833	cholera
1609	Typhus	1853	cholera
1648–54	Yellow Fever, smallpox	1874–75	smallpox
1699	epidemic	1903	yellow fever
1726–27	epidemic	1918–19	influenza
1787	bola		

Sources: Basic information for this table is taken from Farriss, *Maya Society under Colonial Rule*, 61-62, and George Cheever Shattuck, *The Peninsula of Yucatán: Medical, Biological, Meteorological and Sociological Studies* (Washington, DC: Carnegie Institution of Washington, 1933), 336, 338, 340.

fever. Yellow fever arrived in Yucatán shortly after it appeared in Barbados in 1647. It rapidly swept through the Caribbean region, transmitted through the bites of the *Aedes aegypti* mosquito. *Aedes aegypti* likely crossed the Atlantic on slave ships some years earlier and by the 1640s existed in most of the circum-Caribbean region. They certainly found homes in the numerous water casks that were required on every slave ship. The West African home of this mosquito species undermines the claims of some scholars that yellow fever might have arrived with the Spanish, or even that it existed before contact. Survivors of a yellow fever attack are conferred immunity, so that is it quite likely that European sailors and not enslaved Africans hosted the disease in the Atlantic crossing. Like smallpox, a deadly combination of a fast transit and appropriate human hosts brought the disease to the Caribbean.[18]

The yellow fever epidemic began in the port city of Campeche in June 1648.[19] A month later it reached Mérida, where doctors were at a loss to identify the disease. By September it had reached Valladolid, the eastern-most Spanish city in the region. The disease attacked native and colonizer alike, causing terror among the Spanish population. For two years, yellow fever afflicted the region, which was then struck by a crop failure, famine, and, in 1654, smallpox. The combination of disease and famine led to the deaths of perhaps half of the Maya remaining in the lowlands.[20]

Disease and drought-induced famine led to a fluctuating population total during the colonial period. Conquest diseases led to a rapid decline in the population of the region, reaching a low of some 170,000 people around 1580. By 1639, just before yellow fever struck the region, the population had increased to an estimated 222,500 people. Various epidemics and famines over the next century reduced the population to 161,000 people in 1736, after which the total steadily increased. By the end of the colonial period, perhaps half a million people inhabited Yucatán.[21]

DISEASE AND NINETEENTH-CENTURY PUBLIC HEALTH CAMPAIGNS

Knowledge of what *could* be done to fight a disease, ideological conceptions of what *should* be done, and institutional structures shape the capacity to combat disease. Colonial physicians, priests, and *ah-menes* might alleviate emotional and mental suffering, but they could do little to inhibit the physical impact of the great killers, though quarantine and isolation might have offered limited help. Effective public health measures began with the 1803 "Royal Philanthropic Vaccination Expedition," which introduced an operative smallpox vaccine and nascent public health institutions to the region.

Over the nineteenth century, the sanitarian movement and the "Pasteurian Revolution" set the stage for effective disease campaigns.

Methods to prevent smallpox had been known for centuries, but were late in coming to European awareness. Variolation—the transfer of pus from an active pox to another person by a shallow incision in the skin—emerged in China and India in the tenth century, and spread through much of the Muslim world by the seventeenth century. Variolation entered Christian Europe and crossed the Atlantic in the 1720s, though it was not practiced in Mexico until 1779.[22] Jenner's less dangerous vaccination technique created a new public health capacity, leading to the "Royal Philanthropic Vaccination Expedition" (*Expedición Filantrópica de la Vacuna*). Francisco Xavier de Balmis and Dr. Antonio Gutiérrez, one of his principal assistants, taught Dr. Cipriano Blanco how to develop the smallpox vaccine from live pustules. Shortly thereafter, the Yucatec governor ordered the creation of a "Provincial Vaccination Board" to develop and administer the vaccine.[23]

In fits and starts, the anti-smallpox campaign reduced the impact of the disease and contributed to the development of the region's public health infrastructure. Mérida's municipal council and the governor coordinated smallpox vaccination efforts in the state. Political chiefs of the various municipalities would appoint vaccination "subdirectors," who in turn reported to the vaccination director in Mérida, usually a physician at the General Hospital.[24] Subdirectors seldom had access to sufficient quantities of vaccine, and they often encountered popular resistance to vaccinators.[25] None the less, physicians at the School of Medicine, the General Hospital, and the Vaccination Board gained valuable experience, and, perhaps most importantly, contributed to the lessened mortality from the disease.

Less influential than vaccinations were remedies for yellow fever undertaken by the general population of the "destitute and poor classes." Bleeding was reportedly a common treatment for robust patients, especially in the early stages of the disease. Purgatives and laxatives were given at all stages of the disease, while some people lanced the pustules in an effort to forestall their deadly affect. In rural areas, "blistered fever" was treated by the *abal ac e isum che'tamay* root, ground and either applied to the blisters or the tongue.[26] Dr. Francisco Losa y Domínguez, a professor of medicine and a leader in the public health movement, reported that during the 1878–79 epidemic "Indian quacks" amplified the widespread mortality through venesection.[27] Losa's assessment of "popular" medicine enhanced his commitment to a permanent public health agency.

Fortunately, relatively few epidemics afflicted residents of Yucatán in the 1800s. Cholera was the exception. The final epidemic disease to cross the ocean, cholera appeared in Mexico in 1832. The bacteria *Vibrio cholerae* causes severe diarrhea in humans and can lead to dehydration and, within hours, death. Cholera is usually transmitted by drinking water that has been infected by the transfer of bacteria in human feces. It can also be transmitted through food. Though humans host *Vibrio cholerae,* so too do shellfish, in which the bacteria may reside until eaten by humans. Cholera appears to have been endemic to the Indian subcontinent, but burst into six global epidemics beginning in 1817. The epidemic of 1817 did not cross the ocean, but it did in 1831. Within months, the disease spread throughout the US[28] and into Mexico. The disease spread from Cuba into Yucatán in June 1833. Within a month the first cases appeared in Mérida. Physicians associated with the School of Medicine helped combat the disease, whose cause was completely unknown. Fortunately, the epidemic died down within two months, and temporary public health measures were abandoned.[29] A second cholera epidemic reached Yucatán in 1853. Temporary agencies again sought to control the outbreak, and were again abolished when the epidemic ended.

A smallpox outbreak in 1874–75 demonstrated the urgent need for new public health capacities. Physicians in Mérida reported the first case on November 18, when Demetrio Ávila of the barrio San Sebastián sickened. The numbers of deaths quickly increased, leading to the establishment of an asylum to isolate victims of the disease from other patients at the General Hospital. Within one week, at least six people had died, though physicians feared that the number was greater because families were permitted to obtain burial permits without reporting the cause of death.[30] By mid-January 1876, just before the worst stages of the epidemic, some fifty-five people had died.[31] Two weeks later, sixty people a week were dying of the disease in Mérida alone. The February through May period was reportedly the worst of the epidemic.[32] In the end, Mérida reportedly lost 1,637 people; the entire state reported 13,263 deaths.[33] Physicians noted that the epidemic was far worse in the suburbs than in the city, in that inner city residents practiced better hygiene and were more likely to be vaccinated. Death records revealed that of the 116 people who died in the peak weeks in February and March, over ninety percent were under the age of twenty.[34]

Public health officials learned several lessons from this epidemic. First, successful vaccination would have to begin with the youth and must be extended beyond "white" Mérida. Second, the cause of death needed to be determined for each person, and that information needed to be submitted to a permanent, centralized authority. Finally, officials asked that the bodies of smallpox victims should not be exhumed for twice the normal span of two years, because of fears that the disease still might be active.[35] Physician Juan Dondé Ruiz praised local officials for urging that members of the Medical-Pharmaceutical Society draw up a Health Code, but he insisted that public hygiene required a permanent body. This was, Dondé observed, the way "civilized countries" organized their public health organizations. In addition to disease control, such an entity would also carry out sanitary inspections of public establishments.[36]

INTERNATIONAL PUBLIC HEALTH AND TROPICAL MEDICINE

Cholera and yellow fever stimulated the creation of international agencies and new methods to combat easily transmittable diseases. The cholera epidemic of the 1830s led to efforts in Paris (1851) to spur international cooperation to prevent the spread of disease. European and American public health officials periodically met in their respective hemispheres to seek agreements to combat infectious diseases. Quarantine was obviously effective, but its economic repercussions hindered international cooperation. The Eleventh International Sanitary Conference of 1903 produced the "Paris Convention," a foundational document in the regulation of maritime trade and epidemic disease. Four years later the International Office of Public Hygiene was established, to be complemented by the Hygiene Office of the League of Nation in 1920.[37] The 1948 establishment of the World Health Organization of the United Nations continued this tradition, but also undertook more proactive measures to combat diseases.

Conceptions of tropical medicine developed concurrently with international health protocols as imperial powers sought ways to protect the health of their citizens in newly established colonies. Patrick Manson, a British physician working in China, is often credited with associating particular diseases with the tropics. In the 1890s, Manson demonstrated how mosquitoes transferred the *filaria sanguinis hominis* worm that causes elephantiasis,[38] an observation that focused attention on diseases particular to the tropics. Colonial powers quickly developed schools of tropical medicine, such as the London School of Tropical Medicine, where physicians could develop medicines and strategies for dealing with tropical diseases. The Liverpool School of Tropical Medicine, for example, sent out 32 expeditions to the tropics in the fifteen years after its founding in 1899.[39]

In the Americas, yellow fever was the leading "tropical disease." A range of scholars played critical roles in bringing yellow fever under control. Cuban Carlos Finlay isolated the *Culex* mosquito (*Aedes Aegypti*) as the transmitter of the disease in the 1880s, but his breakthrough attracted little attention. In tracing the spread of yellow fever in a Mississippi outbreak, Henry Rose Carter concluded in 1898 against direct transmission of the disease and for the existence of an intermediate host. During the US occupation of Cuba, Jesse Lazear confirmed the *Culex* as the host, subjecting himself to the bites of the mosquito—with fatal results. Walter Reed, a member of the US Yellow

Fever Commission, and William C. Gorgas, a Cuban working with Reed, attacked the mosquito in Havana with militarized precision. Open waters were drained, covered with a layer of oil to suffocate the larvae, or seeded with larvae-eating fish. Door-to-door campaigns used similar tactics, and urged that residents use mosquito netting over their beds. Cases of yellow fever and malaria declined dramatically.[40] The US Army Yellow Fever Commission, the US Public Health and Marine Hospital Service (USPHS), the Rockefeller Foundation, and national public health officials used these tactics to eliminate the threat of yellow fever from the upper Caribbean region and much of Latin America over the next two decades.

The ability to control yellow fever through sanitation methods spurred international cooperation. Delegates from fifteen countries attended the Second International Conference of the American States in Mexico City (1901–02). The meeting produced plans for the International Sanitary Bureau (1902), an organization with hemispheric responsibilities. In time, this agency would become the Pan American Health Organization (PAHO). Tensions over the economic impact of quarantines persisted, especially as Latin American nations did not have officials in US ports, as the USPHS had in many of theirs.[41] Although productive meetings were held in Rio de Janeiro (1906) and Mexico City (1907), a sanitary code for the Americas was not adopted until the seventh conference held in Havana, in November 1924; this code was intended to prevent international spread of disease, coordinate quarantine efforts, and create uniform procedures among member states.[42]

TWENTIETH-CENTURY PUBLIC HEALTH CAMPAIGNS

The late nineteenth-century conjunction of new medical knowledge and technologies, permanent public health agencies, and patterns of international cooperation transformed public health campaigns in Yucatán. The *Junta Superior de Sanidad* attended to a variety of diseases, as well as sanitation, food and water quality, prostitution, and the hygienic inspection of public facilities. Federal authorities and international agencies became increasingly active in the same period, so that Yucatec officials often interacted with Mexican officials and international partners. Despite these new developments—but more often as a result—tensions between the state and federal governments, and resistance by Yucatec residents persisted into the new century.

Public health campaigns followed two broad patterns in twentieth-century Yucatán. Campaigns against epidemic diseases such as smallpox, yellow fever, and malaria continued with increased national and international cooperation. A variety of factors led to the reduced frequency of epidemics, so that the 1918 influenza outbreak proved to be the last of the great killers to afflict the region. The second pattern dealt with more localized concerns, such as improving sanitary conditions, the regulation of prostitution, or combating rabies. Local officials proved largely indifferent to rural problems, and tended to ignore those who argued for a focus upon illnesses with a social origin. As the federal government instituted revolutionary health care programs beginning in the 1930s, federal officials came to dominate local efforts. By the late 1950s, federal and state officials more often worked in tandem, with national health organizations clearly in positions of authority.

Smallpox

The smallpox vaccination campaign received added support with the creation of the *Junta Superior*. In 1889, the state government mandated that all residents be vaccinated, but a shortage of vaccine and vaccinators frustrated that objective.[43] The Vaccination Board maintained regular contact with vaccinators in local towns, usually priests or members of the town council. Typical of the management effort was a July 1891 note to the *jefe político* of Ticul asking for a list of those who had been vaccinated, and an estimate of how many tubes of vaccine would be needed to complete the task.[44] The task became somewhat easier with the establishment of the *Junta Superior*, as it could appoint physicians to replace poorly performing vaccinators.

Yucatec officials developed new methods in the ongoing campaign against smallpox that would influence campaigns against other diseases. Initially, vaccination efforts constituted the primary thrust of the campaign, just as they had in the nineteenth century. The *Junta Superior de Sanidad* reported the numbers of persons who had been vaccinated with obvious pride, though it reported problems as well.[45] In 1894, for example, the *Junta* reported that 1,225 people had been vaccinated in Mérida, almost three percent of the city's population. In the state, however, only 2,103 people had been vaccinated. This shortfall allegedly stemmed from the perennial problem of obtaining sufficient vaccine, but also the "lack of enlightenment" in areas removed from "civilization and progress." This clear reference to the Mayan interior reflected the sensibilities of the white elite of the capital city. The *Junta Superior* urged Governor Carlos Peón to require mandatory vaccinations of all persons under ten, an edit that he issued in 1895.[46] *Jefes políticos* reported that recruiting clergy or *hacendados* to assist the campaign offered the greatest opportunity of success, as the natives themselves looked upon the campaign with "indifference."[47] By 1902, sixty vaccination centers operated in the state's interior, offering monthly inoculations. Residents of Mérida could receive inoculations daily.[48]

An adequate supply of vaccine continued to hamper the campaign. A small outbreak in 1903 redoubled the urgency of sufficient doses. Supplies from

Mexico City could not satisfy the need, so that the *Junta* turned first to the Pasteur Institute in New York City and then to the Pasteur headquarters in Paris.[49] Increased supplies, much of it produced locally by the *Junta*, and vaccination management produced positive results. Between 1893 and 1907 over 256,000 people were vaccinated, perhaps three-quarters of the state's population.[50]

The anti-smallpox campaign included the port of Progreso. One of the first actions of the *Junta Superior* was to focus upon the vaccination of all persons who worked on the docks or came into contact with visitors.[51] The forced movement of Yaqui Indians to labor in Yucatán's henequen haciendas exacerbated problems within the anti-smallpox campaign. Unvaccinated Yaqui laborers, it was thought, would make smallpox epidemics more likely. Thus, in the midst of a minor outbreak in 1908, the *Junta* suggested that all immigrants be detained in Progreso until they were vaccinated. Asian migrants would be inspected for trachoma in the same method.[52] As a result, when 112 Yaquis arrived at the port in March, *Junta* officials sent vaccine to the coast to inoculate them all.[53]

New organizational strategies complemented the ongoing vaccination effort.[54] Dr. José Montes de Oca reported in April 20, 1915 that he had found a case of smallpox in Motul while investigating an outbreak of measles. The *Junta* mobilized auxiliary health brigades in towns affected by the disease, a campaign assisted by revolutionary troops under Salvador Alvarado.[55] Local brigades were led by students from the School of Medicine, who would be in charge of vaccinations. Victims would either be isolated locally or sent to Mérida for treatment; their houses would be disinfected. All persons in the community would be revaccinated. Anyone found harboring a smallpox victim would be subject to a 100-peso fine.[56] Prompt isolation and wholesale vaccination procedures appeared to be effective, as only 20,750 cases were reported in Yucatán in 1915, a small percentage of the population that then exceeded 300,000.[57]

The 1917 expansion of the *Junta Superior de Sanidad* included substantial laboratory improvement. This seemingly enabled the organization to finally satisfy its own demand for vaccine. Governor Alvaro Torre Díaz reported an 85 percent success rate of vaccination during his term in office (1926–30). No case of smallpox appeared in the state throughout the 1920s.[58]

Yellow Fever

Disease and trade patterns helped shape the Upper Caribbean, a maritime region bounded by Mexico, the United States, and Cuba. Extensive trading relations linked the major ports of Havana, New Orleans, and Veracruz, as well as Yucatán's primary port of Progreso.[59] The fear of the transmission of cholera, yellow fever, and malaria led to cooperation—and antagonisms—among port officials of the region. Agents of the USPHS stationed in Progreso monitored all ships coming or going from the port, kept commercial records, inspected patents, and disinfected ships.[60] Mexican federal public health officials maintained a delegation in the port, as did state authorities. In the 1890s, the Progreso *jefe politico* decided that a commission of these public health delegates should determine if a particular boat needed to be quarantined, a move that the United States rejected, favoring autonomy of decision-making.[61]

The cause of yellow fever was unknown when the *Junta Superior* was founded. Physicians knew that newcomers to the region were highly susceptible to the disease. Long-time residents were much less likely to fall victim to its periodic outbreaks. Monitoring the port of Progreso seemingly limited the flow of the disease from the Upper Caribbean, especially from Havana, a yellow fever hotspot. In Mérida, isolation of victims and fumigation of their houses, both sanitarian methods, were common responses to the disease. In rural areas, the thatched *na* of victims was often burned, as its design prevented effective fumigation.

The *Junta Superior* used these methods in response to the 1903 outbreak of yellow fever in the Dzitás region east of Mérida. In his initial report, W. G. Cantón reported that some 70 members of the "indigenous race" were suffering from the disease. Cantón speculated that heavy rains in the region produced widespread standing water that allowed for a large population of mosquitoes, so that the outbreak was likely to be more localized than widespread. By the end of the month, six people had died, and victims were being admitted to an asylum in Mérida for isolation and treatment. The outbreak ebbed by the end of the year, with the Mérida asylum reporting 172 admissions, 67 of who succumbed to the disease.[62]

The anti-larval methods developed in Havana took several years to reach Yucatán, and then were implemented under federal rather than state auspices. The success of the Reed campaign in Havana stimulated the Mexican government to launch a drive against yellow fever in 1903. Though the campaign began in the Vera cruz region, federal health chief Eduardo Liceaga dispatched sanitation brigades to Campeche and Yucatán in 1905. In Campeche, sanitary brigades drained and oiled swamps to destroy the habitat of the mosquito that transmitted the disease, and ordered the mandatory use of quinine, a treatment method known for centuries.[63]

Federal sanitary delegates Pedro Medina V. and José Lavalle A. arrived in the Yucatec capital in August 1906 to launch the program in Mérida. Following the pattern employed in Vera cruz, Mérida was divided into four quarters, each under the supervision of a physician and supported by various agents. Federal agents also operated in Progreso.[64] Intensive house-to-house inspections began in May 1908, revealing many open cisterns, even though a 1904 state statute had ordered that water systems be covered. Federal delegates and *Junta* officials ordered countless residents to cap their cisterns within fifteen days or face a hefty fine.[65] From this time until the end of the federal program in 1911, local officials regularly informed Mexico City of all cases of yellow fever.[66] As the Revolution brought the federal campaign to a close, local physician Gil Rojas Aguilar was named a federal sanitary delegate and continued the effort to limit the breeding grounds of the *Aedes aegypti* mosquito.

Yucatec physicians and others often speculated as to whether or not members of the Maya population were immune to yellow fever. Alonso Avila E., for example, read a paper on the topic at a January 1906 meeting of the "Arcadia" society. Avila suggested that while yellow fever was not common among the Maya, the 1878 and 1903 outbreaks convinced him that they were susceptible. "Natives" (either of the indigenous race or mestizos) and whites who had lived in the region for a long time were comparably susceptible.[67] After an outbreak in 1911, Diego Hernández Fajardo seconded Avila's conclusions at a meeting of the Yucatec Medical Society, suggesting a consensus among local physicians that indigenous populations were in no way immune from the disease, though they did not contract the disease as easily.[68] (It is likely that they must have contracted milder cases in childhood and development immunity.)

Newcomers to the peninsula, by contrast, routinely contracted yellow fever. Soldiers and merchants were often victims. In 1881, for example, the Military Hospital in Mérida reported 41 cases among the 500 soldiers in the city; twenty-one succumbed to the disease.[69] Seventy-three people contracted the disease in 1911–12, most of whom were soldiers who had recently arrived from the interior of Mexico. That outbreak claimed thirty-eight lives, a death rate of just over fifty percent.[70]

Just as the federal government withdrew from the region in 1911, yellow fever again broke out. Physician and Governor Nicolás Cámara Vales invited Harald Seidelin to return to Yucatán to investigate the disease. Seidelin, it will be remembered, had lived in Mérida for four years (1906–10), developing the laboratory facilities of the Hospital O'Horán and School of Medicine. Seidelin's objective for this visit (December 29, 1911–May 27, 1912) was the isolation of the germ of the disease.[71] Seidelin thought that the *Paraplasma flavigenum* bore a special relationship to yellow fever. He looked for *paraplasma* in dozens of water samples taken throughout the city and region. He found instead the presence of *Stegomyia fasciata* in almost 80 percent of the samples from all areas of the city and rural areas. Predictably, open water cisterns housed the larvae, as did sewer water collected at intersections. His microscopic studies of the disease failed to isolate the yellow fever germ.[72]

Seidelin and laboratory specialist Rafael Betancourt Agramonte also focused upon the nature of the disease among multiple populations. Seidelin adhered to the theory that Mérida and Yucatán had hosted the disease since pre-Columbian days. Indigenous locals contracted the disease early in life, manifesting relatively benign cases. Spaniards who lived in the region for a long period experienced the same pattern. Adult newcomers manifested virulent cases, often ending in their death. In any case, Seidelin and Betancourt confirmed Avila's suspicion of Maya susceptibility to the disease. Maya residents of Motul suffered various cases of the disease in 1912. Seidelin brought several ill residents of Kambul, a few kilometers to the west of Motul, to the lazaretto of the capital to be treated. Unfortunately, several people died of the disease, enabling Seidelin and Betancourt Agramonte to confirm the yellow fever diagnosis by postmortem analysis.[73]

Seidelin criticized years of anti-yellow fever campaigns as largely inefficient. To be sure, progress had been made, but much more work remained. *Junta* officials needed to attend cisterns more aggressively, though he thought that only an underground water and sewer system would remove breeding locations. Areas where insects bred needed to be filled, as he saw oiling as a less effective treatment. Open air fumigation should be used in urban areas.[74] Seidelin returned to England before his suggestions were fully implemented, though Gil Rojas worked aggressively on them during the 1910s.

The last case of yellow fever in Yucatán occurred in 1920, just as the Rockefeller Foundation sought permission to extend to Mexico its campaign against the disease. After intensive negotiations, the International Health Board (IHB) of the Rockefeller Foundation joined the Mexican government in the Special Commission for the Eradication of yellow Fever (1921–24), with one regional center in Mérida. Rockefeller activities in Yucatán have attracted the attention of numerous scholars, adding to an abundant scholarship on the organization that served as the eventual model for the World Health Organization.[75]

In 1919, Rockefeller laboratory scientist Hideyo Noguchi made an apparent breakthrough in Guayaquil, Ecuador—the development of a yellow fever vaccine.[76] This led to feverish diplomatic activity and an invitation from the Mexican government that Noguchi visit Mérida to treat a small outbreak of the fever. Noguchi arrived in Mérida shortly before Christmas 1919 to a hero's welcome. The *Revista Médica de Yucatán* headlined their January 1920 edition "Noguchi in Yucatán," reprinting his report from Guayaquil. A major conference at the Hospital O'Horán led the School of Medicine to name him an honorary member, an induction witnessed by most of Mérida's public health community.[77]

The *Junta Superior de Sanidad* opened their new laboratory for Noguchi's use, where he worked closely with its director, Abelardo Lara. Noguchi soon located *Leptospira icteroides* and began to produce vaccine and serum.[78] After only a few weeks, Noguchi left Yucatán for New York, and then continued on to a research campaign in Peru.[79] The *Junta* continued his labors, administering the vaccine to 3,477 people, most of them members of the military, but also to some local residents.[80] Director Rojas Aguilar traveled to New York later that year to obtain more vaccine, a request Noguchi was pleased to grant, though he asked Yucatec officials to closely monitor reactions to the vaccine.[81] Though other scientists failed to reproduce Noguchi's results, including those at the Rockefeller Center, Noguchi published several papers on his vaccine before his death in 1928 due to of yellow fever in the Gold Coast.[82] In the end, the vaccine was ineffective.

The Special Commission began its efforts in early 1921, led by M. E. Connor in Yucatán. The IHB insisted upon an "intensive" anti-larval approach that began with the construction of a detailed map of Mérida, noting each house, commercial enterprise, public building, and source of water. Connor divided Mérida into eleven districts, with each house inspected over ten-day period. Inspectors would then meet to report on issues in their zones and decide upon strategies to pursue in the subsequent rounds.[83] Rojas Aguilar and his eleven-man team undertook an impressive range of activities in the campaign. In November 1921, for example, they performed 33,671 house visits, examined 136,059 water deposits (they oiled, emptied, or fished 41,298 of the deposits), and found 12,055 larvae.[84] As the campaign ended in 1924, 14 agents, 16 helpers, and 2 "tank sealers" were laboring in the capital.[85] Progreso operated as a single zone; as in Mérida, state officials dominated the Commission's activities, with little apparent cooperation with federal maritime officials at the port.[86]

With the last reported case of yellow fever in Mexico in December 1922, Connor confidently predicted that the Special Commission would end its work. Given a year without the disease, he proposed ending the campaign on November 30, 1923. Both federal officials and the IHB appeared satisfied with the date, which would herald the inauguration of a campaign against hookworm.[87] The Special Commission justly claimed credit for helping to eliminate yellow fever from Mexico, though in Yucatán the claim might be overstated.

The incidence of yellow fever in Yucatán had declined rapidly in the first decades of the twentieth century, with the last case in 1920. Connor envisioned several factors for the decline. The disease had become endemic in the henequen zone in the late nineteenth century, with migratory laborers the most frequent victims. Connor thought that the decline of henequen in the 1910s reduced the pool of potential victims. Further, as steamships replaced sailing ships, there were fewer opportunities for the passage of the mosquito. Finally, the Havana anti-mosquito campaign had broken the "vicious cycle" of transmission in the major Caribbean ports.[88]

Local physician Pedro F. Rivas offered a somewhat different analysis. Rivas argued that rather than declining, the numbers of imported laborers increased in the 1910s and the numbers of federal troops rose dramatically. The sanitary actions by the Junta *Superior* and federal government had brought the disease under control prior to the arrival of the Special Commission.[89] Ana María Carrillo agrees upon the importance of early anti-yellow fever efforts, though with more emphasis upon federal rather than state responsibility.[90] The effective operations of Yucatán's *Junta Superior de Sanidad* facilitated the work of both the 1903 and 1921 campaigns. State and federal efforts eliminated the disease, but the 1921 commission no doubt worked against its recurrence. The human and organizational infrastructures were well-prepared to cooperate with both Mexican and IHB officials, bringing the dreaded disease under control.

Anti-larval techniques continued in both Mérida and Progreso after the Special Commission came to a conclusion. In defending the ongoing campaign in the midst of budget cuts in 1924, Federal Sanitary Delegate Hernández reported that it would be impossible to reduce the number of people working for the service. The 14 inspectors, 16 helpers, and 2 seal inspectors were necessary to conduct the weekly inspection system instituted by Connor.[91] Charles E. Athey, an agent of the US Public Health Service stationed in Progreso, noted that agents from both the federal Maritime Sanitary Service and Yucatec *Servicio Antilavario* were active in the port. In 1926 four teams scoured the city, examining pools of standing water, cisterns, and sanitary facilities. The teams would empty vessels with standing water, pour oil onto pools of water, or place fish in cisterns to eat the larvae.[92] Fortunately, some of these methods affected the incidences of malaria as well.

Malaria

By the 1910s, the nature and transmission of malaria was well-known, though the disease would prove far harder to eradicate than yellow fever. The seventeenth-century discovery of cinchona bark (quinine) allowed for the control of the *calenturas* (fevers) caused by the disease,[93] but not its elimination. Charles Louis Alphonse Laveran isolated *plasmodium* in malaria sufferers in 1882. Italian research Camillo Golgi determined that different types of malaria existed caused by different types of the *plasmodium*, creating "urban" and "jungle" versions of the disease. The anti-larval methods used against yellow fever assisted in the control of the urban disease, but was less effective in controlling the disease in the interior, as the mosquitoes did not need humans to transmit the *plasmodium*, and had a far more extensive habitat.

Malaria ranked lower on the public health agenda than smallpox or yellow fever, despite the fact that most communities suffered from the disease. Outbreaks of the disease were common, such as a March 1923 episode in Progreso that afflicted some 700 of the town's 10,000 residents.[94] In 1922, the municipal council of Hocobá reported that forty percent of the residents were sickened by the disease. Governor Carrillo Puerto replied that he would dispatch medical brigades from the *Liga de Resistencia* to the community, and would alert public health officials of the problem.[95] Rojas Aguilar complained to the governor in early 1922 that a shortage of funds had limited the campaign to yellow fever, when malaria was widespread in the state.[96] Fortunately, these brief epidemics had comparatively low mortality rates; during a 1925–26 outbreak in Mérida 2.4 percent of the victims lost their lives.[97]

The anti-yellow fever infrastructure was reoriented to attack malaria after 1924. After a severe epidemic in 1927 in Progreso, the federal public health officer Carlos C. Hoffman joined *Junta* delegate Román Sabas Flores in investigating the disease. The disease was concentrated in the workers' neighborhood "Francisco I. Madero," a district located next to the marshes. Poor sanitation conditions and unusual levels of rainfall spurred the epidemic, which killed scores of residents. Cooperation by agents of DSP, the federal Maritime Delegation (*Delegación Sanitaria Marítima*), and both state and federal anti-larvae services fought the disease. Their studies found the *Anopheles* in 92 percent of houses. Their primary treatment was fumigation using "Flit," which had been imported from New Orleans. Groups of four soldiers under direction of health service workers emptied an "infected" house, covered furniture, and then set off the fumigating bomb. The agents also undertook anti-larval activities, drainage, and oiling to control the mosquito. Hoffman and Sabas Flores urged that the aggressive campaign be extended throughout the state, though they acknowledged both a shortage of quinine and resources would hinder that effort.[98]

The federal *Servicio de Enfermedades Tropicales* (Tropical Disease Service) conducted most anti-malaria services in the state. It maintained seventeen posts in 1930, though a shortage of funds led to a cession of oiling in Mérida, with similar reductions elsewhere.[99] The campaign was transferred to the jurisdiction of Rural Hygiene and Social Medicine in 1948, when 1,525 cases were active.[100] When the Rockefeller Foundation joined forces with the Mexican government to combat the disease in the 1950s, the campaign was not active in Yucatán,[101] leaving residents to suffer as they had for years.

Influenza

The influenza pandemic of 1918–1919 took the lives of at least 50 million people worldwide. The disease reached Yucatán in late 1918. As the nature of the epidemic became clearer, Rojas Aguilar convinced the governor to ban all public festivals during the duration of the outbreak. The January 24 ban extended to upcoming Carnival events, Holy Week activities, and even to school celebrations.[102] The auxiliary units organized during the 1915 smallpox outbreak were put into action, especially in interior towns. The *Junta Superior de Sanidad* ordered medical students and physicians into the countryside in response to the outbreaks, with orders to quarantine and treat the ill.

A regular stream of correspondence describing horrific conditions flowed into Mérida. Tizimín reportedly had some of the worst conditions in the state. Dr. Ermilo Samperio arrived in Tizimín to find 1,800 sick people; he ran out of supplies in less than 48 hours. Director Rojas Aguilar dispatched two nurses, two students, and supplies to assist the beleaguered physician.[103] Medical student Enrique Díaz reported that he had treated 135 people in the town of Chablekal in the last week of January. Sixty appeared to have recovered, seventy were still sick, and five people succumbed to the disease.[104] Much to his relief, Samperio reported in late February that the worst of the outbreak appeared to have passed. Agents in Sucilá, Calotmul, Abalá, Chablekal, Ixil, Ramón, Carranca, and Kixkokob observed that the disease had peaked by February in their areas. In March, *La Higiene* reported that in the four months since the beginning of the epidemic, some 100,000 people had been examined in the state, and that five people had lost their lives each day in the worst phases of the epidemic.[105] The JSS declared the influenza epidemic over in April.[106] Mérida suffered 1,460 deaths in the epidemic; 3,221 people died statewide.[107]

Prostitution

Governments throughout the Atlantic community legalized prostitution in the nineteenth century, principally as a means to control the spread of venereal disease. The Yucatec government legalized prostitution in 1881, a process that became deeply institutionalized with the establishment of the *Junta Superior*. Anti-prostitution efforts in Yucatán were initially justified as a means to control the spread of venereal disease, but Revolutionary leaders such as Salvador Alvarado and Carrillo Puerto suggested that regulation had positive moral consequences as well.[108]

The *ayuntamiento* of Mérida took the initial steps to regulate prostitution. The 1881 edict required that prostitutes register with the *jefe político*, work only in approved houses, and submit to regular medical inspections. Bordellos required at least two women to be managed by a madam, and only in certain zones of the city.[109] Women who failed to register and continued to sell sexual services became "clandestine prostitutes" and were liable to legal persecution.[110]

The organization of the *Junta Superior de Sanidad* created a public health infrastructure to supervise prostitution throughout the state. All municipal organizations were required to report prostitution to the *Junta*, who would monitor registered prostitutes. The 1896 Sanitary Code made notable changes regarding prostitution: women would now need to pay a two and one-half peso registration fee to the JSS, and a similar monthly payment to cover their inspections; solo prostitutes would now be permitted outside the bordellos. Only single women over the age of fifteen would be permitted to prostitute themselves; married women or widows could not sell their bodies.[111] A 1903 modification of the sanitary code increased to ten pesos the registration fee for prostitutes and to 100 pesos for houses. House owners also had to pay a 100-peso fee for health inspections.[112] In keeping with these statutes, for example, Caridad Beritán was granted the right to serve as a *pupila* at the house No. 603 on Calle 61.[113]

Monitoring the healthiness of prostitutes occupied significant energies. Women were supposed to appear for weekly examinations. Different staff members were responsible for one week of gynecological exams every month. In October 1908, for example, Arturo Erosa covered the first week, followed by Romualdo Manjarrez and Waldemaro G. Cantón.[114] When women such as María Cruz Hernández Ruis failed to report for her January 14 appointment, she was fined five pesos and told to report to the Hospital O'Horán for treatment.[115] Vocales reported a case of clandestine prostitution in June 1899, asking that the *jefe político* fine the owner of the house ten pesos, and the same amount to both women who had not properly registered.[116] In a six-month period in 1902, prostitution inspectors received 2,757.65 pesos in fees and reported 76 cases of infectious diseases.[117]

Some critics argued that both prostitution and venereal diseases increased during periods of poor economic conditions. Yucatán suffered an economic shock at the end of World War I as demand for henequen declined. Women would migrate to the city to earn a living prostituting themselves, leading to an increase in prostitution.[118] In September 1922, 73 women were registered with JSS.[119] In spite of alleged revolutionary empathy with poor women forced into prostitution, neither Alvarado nor Carrillo Puerto took steps to criminalize the activity. Critics maintained that regulation expanded the numbers of prostitutes, giving social sanction to activities that were socially detrimental. This logic led Governor Torre Díaz to end the legalization experiment in 1927.[120] It is likely that legal prostitution failed to significantly reduce the rate of venereal diseases in Mérida, just as it failed in Buenos Aires and elsewhere.[121]

Rabies

As early as 1875 the *ayuntamiento* of Mérida had initiated a strategy of combating rabies by killing "street dogs." Town officials placed poison in small bits of meat, giving it to dogs that ran free and did not have a collar. Owners were urged to use collars with their addresses on their dogs, or face the possibility of their dogs being poisoned. One observer noted that the results of the campaign were "painful to see," and that the bodies were often left on the street to decompose. Predictably, the campaign focused on the center of the city, where more affluent people lived, rather than in the poorer (and indigenous) suburbs. Periodic publication of the description of rabies symptoms accompanied the anti-street dog campaign.[122]

While praising the labor of the *ayuntamiento*, José Ricardo Saurí reported shortcomings in their efforts. First, the campaign had to be permanent. Within three years after regulations were enacted, Suarí noted that they were infrequently enforced. Moreover, they had little effect on dogs in indigenous communities, where rabies was allegedly more common. Suarí claimed that the pants of indigenous men, which ended just below the knee, made dog bites and the transmission of the disease more likely.[123] He did not, however, suggest a possible solution to the problem.

Changing medical technology enabled a distinct approach to the anti-rabies campaign. After Louis Pasteur and Émile Roux developed a vaccine against the disease in 1885, Yucatec officials had a second tool for controlling rabies. The vaccine could be made locally by infecting a rabbit and allowing it to develop the disease. The animal would then be killed and its spinal cord removed and allowed to dry. A small portion of the cord would be injected into a person bitten by a rabid animal, with high degrees of success. Given this technology, the effort to end rabies in Yucatán involved two distinct sets of activities, one preventative and the other reactive. Preventative measures focused on the effort to eliminate "street dogs." Dogs were not supposed to run loose, were to wear labeled collars, and owners were supposed to muzzle dogs that were not restrained. Poisoning of dogs constituted the second leg of the preventative effort.[124] The reactive phase involved the treatment of anyone bitten by a dog. Public officials, especially police officers in Mérida and *jefes politicos* in the interior, were asked to report all bites and to immediately capture the dog for shipment to the capital. The victim would accompany the animal to receive the rabies vaccine. Though the vaccine was free, kenneling the dog was to be paid by the owner.

The *Junta Superior* opened a laboratory dedicated to the production of the rabies vaccine in 1912. Gustavo Vega headed the lab, which was supported by mandatory vaccinations according to the sanitary code.[125] Insofar as the reactive phase of the campaign required both laboratory and kennel facilities, an expanded laboratory was included in the new 1917 building.[126]

The campaign against street dogs accelerated in the 1920s. In this phase of the campaign, the *Junta* developed a partnership with *ayuntamientos* or town councils throughout the state. In the 1926–30 gubernatorial period of Torre

Díaz, over a thousand people were treated by the Anti-Rabies Service, 891 dogs were monitored (50 were rabid), and almost 700 rabbits were used to develop the vaccine. Torre Díaz proudly reported that no one who had been vaccinated in these years developed the disease.[127]

The killing of dogs accelerated as well. Strychnine was the preferred poison. *Junta* officials in Mérida frequently reminded local officials that strychnine pills were best placed in small bits of tripe at the last minute, as dogs would otherwise refuse the offered tidbits. In 1934, *Junta* officials complained to the governor that their 200 peso monthly budget did not meet their expenses, especially as public health officials in Campeche made ready use of their services, and that owner fines, kennel fees, and the cost of strychnine pills were seldom paid on time.[128] By 1949, officials killed 3,854 street dogs in Mérida, while 782 met their demise in the interior. Almost 2,500 vaccinations were administered to those who had been bitten.[129]

The anti-rabies campaign illustrates the union of public health infrastructure and capacity. The development of the Pasteur vaccine coincided with the desire to limit the range of street dogs. With the creation of the *Junta Superior*, the campaign became one of the most consistent public health activities in the state. (Sanitary inspections and anti-rabies activities occupied two-thirds of the *Junta*'s actions after 1924. See Table 2.1, chapter 2.) It is unclear whether the incidences of rabies declined, or the numbers of street dogs were reduced. The campaign, however, extended a public health presence throughout the state, even if it had uncertain health consequences.

Tuberculosis

Although tuberculosis is an ancient disease, recognition of the breadth of its presence in Yucatán developed only slowly. The *Junta Superior de Sanidad* collected information on cases of tuberculosis, but did little to fight the disease. Yucatán did not join the sanitarium movement, the widespread process whereby sufferers of tuberculosis were confined to sanitariums, a treatment that lessened its contagious spread among the general population, but which did little to affect a cure among its sufferers.[130] Sufferers might be admitted to Asilo Ayala, but more often they stayed at home. Robert Koch isolated the bacillus *Mycobacterium tuberculosis* in 1882, but not until the 1920s was a general vaccine (BCG) broadly administered. X-ray machines and microscopic studies revealed the disease. Antibiotics proved to be an effective method of treatment after the end of the Second World War, though drug-resistant strains of the bacillus have made eradication of the disease quite problematic.[131] As these detection and treatment methods became widely assessable, officials initiated anti-tuberculosis campaigns.

Physicians associated with the *Sociedad Médica Yucateca* recognized tuberculosis as a "social disease" that required distinct methods of control. In 1905, Dr. Alvaro Avila E. asserted that the campaigns against smallpox and yellow fever had largely been won, but that social diseases would require a distinct type of public health campaign. Avila urged that tuberculosis needed to be combated through the youth. Education in the schools and home would enable the youth to establish healthy patterns that might prevent the disease. Avila suggested that though research indicated that TB was not hereditary, it did have a predisposition toward families of alcoholics and syphilitics, and it was strongly correlated with poor hygienic conditions. Public education, again, could serve as a good preventative. Improved public sanitation was a critical step to attack this social disease. Bars, barbershops, and—especially—houses of prostitution needed to be inspected on a regular basis.[132] Though others joined Avila in calling for a new public health agenda, there is little indication that the *Junta* altered its activities to address this or other "social diseases."

Harald Seidilin and his laboratory associates at the Hospital O'Horán documented the extent of tuberculosis in Mérida. They conducted 146 autopsies in 1909, "most of them" with signs of tuberculosis. Additional bacteriological investigations of 411 suspected cases yielded 184 positive results. In an effort to determine the origins of the disease, A. Erosa and Francisco Colomé worked with local veterinarians to survey the region's cattle ranches. They suggested two actions: develop relations with local vets and the establishment of new regulations to control the spread of the disease from cows to humans.[133] Seidelin concluded that tuberculosis might be the most common disease in Mérida, with an estimated 3,531 cases among the city's 60,000 residents between 1905 and 1909.[134]

Revolutionary agrarian programs might have aggravated the problem of tuberculosis in Yucatán. The rigid isolation of laborers on henequen plantations, and the tendency of families in the corn zone to stay close to their villages meant that the highly contagious disease was less easily spread. Henequen laborers gained more mobility with the establishment of *ejidos* in the 1930s; so too did the disease.[135] The tendency to move to Mérida undoubtedly contributed to the increased numbers of diseased individuals. For Dr. Eduardo Aguilar Gómez, this indicated that diseases that accompanied the misery and hunger of the "humble people and *campesinos* of Yucatán" were noticed only when they began to affect the middle classes, and only when physicians pursued a program of revolutionary health care.[136]

A federal campaign against the disease developed in the 1930s. Data from Mérida indicated only sixteen deaths annually in 1934–35, no doubt seriously undercounting the extent of the disease. Federal Sanitary Delegates began their anti-tuberculosis campaign the next year, funded in part by a one centavo tax on alcohol. The *Servicio Antituberculoso* (Anti-Tuberculosis Service) in Mérida created the first anti-tuberculosis dispensary in Yucatán, diagnosing an average of 204 cases annually in the capital city. A second dispensary was constructed in Progreso in 1942.[137] By 1940, the federal infrastructure to combat tuberculosis was well developed. The Federal Sanitary Delegation managed the campaign with three doctors; twenty-seven nurses dealt with various sanitary illnesses.[138]

In time, the federal and state governments cooperated in the campaign against tuberculosis. Sufferers from the countryside were sent to the *Hospital O'Horán* to receive treatment. Unfortunately, confinement at the hospital did little to treat the disease. Of the 1,686 cases diagnosed at the hospital between 1935 and 1944, 817 sufferers died of the disease.[139] After 1946, ASHOY clinics in the henequen zone used a mobile X-Ray machine to aid in the detection of the disease. In its initial examinations, the "Picker" machine caused "great surprise" by revealing higher rates of the disease than expected.[140] Tuberculosis persisted as a serious disease and declined only with the development of specific drugs, medical attentiveness, and the public health system, variables that came together only after World War II.

WATER, GASTROINTESTINAL DISEASES, AND INFANT MORTALITY

Water-borne gastrointestinal diseases affected the whole of the state. They accounted for high rates of infant mortality, but many adults also died of dysentery or other illness associated with poor water quality. The karst topography of the region limited access to water to *cenotes*, wells, and rainwater stored in underground cisterns (*aljibes*). Thousands of windmills drawing water from the shallow aquifer defined Mérida's early twentieth-century skyline, wells that were often contaminated by human wastes. The paving of streets in the center of the city in the 1910s amplified run off problems during the thunderstorms of the rainy season. Contaminated water supplies increased gastrointestinal diseases in those periods.[141]

Urban progress "naturally" outpaced changes in rural water systems. Olegario Molina spurred the modernization with bold projects, including the paving of downtown streets and the installation of a water and sewer system.[142] These efforts did little to improve the quality of Mérida's water. George Burnell, the general manager of the Mérida Water Company, reported in 1924 that most residents used rainwater or wells, with only a small minority drawing water from the city water system. Burnell noted the high quality of water stored from rain, but observed that it was often contaminated by sediments and bird excretions from rooftops or cisterns.

Water drawn from the aquifer by wells or windmills was by far of the lowest quality. Writing of the governor's house, Burnell reported that "this water is absolutely unfit for drinking purposes and contains a great deal of sewage affluent and harmful germ live."[143] The water from the Grand Hotel was the "worse received from Mérida and is a positive menace to health."[144] Twenty years later, little had improved. Over half of the city's houses were not connected to the sewage system, using privies in their courtyards. There remained over 20,000 wells, drawing upon the "black waters" of the subsoils under the city.[145]

Rural waters were equally poor. The Carnegie report estimated that during the 1926–29 period, between 35 and 45 percent of all deaths in Valladolid, Dzitas, Mérida, Ticul, Peto, and Progreso could be linked to poor water quality.[146] Writing in *La Revista Médica de Yucatán*, two physicians illustrated the breadth of the peninsula's gastrointestinal crisis in a 1946 study. Santiago Leal Arcero and Alfonso Albertos Tenorio collected information from the social assistance program of the *Henequeneros de Yucatán*, the Hospital O'Horán, the *Hospital del Niño*, the federal sanitary delegation, and private laboratories of Hernández Fajardo and René Peniche Cantón. Intestinal parasites figured to be the "major pathogen" of the region, affecting "all sexes, all ages, and all social classes" in "all regions of the state."[147]

High rates of infant mortality were directly linked to water quality. A September 1911 Yucatec Medical Society discussion focused upon the social agenda of many European and Latin American governments. Nearly twice as many infants died each year in Mérida than in Havana, even though the Cuban capital had double the population.[148] In December 1923, Alberto Berrón Guerrero, a leading spokesman for the *Sociedad Médica Yucateca*, lamented that infant mortality had increased, especially among the proletariat.[149] By 1941, twenty-one percent of Mérida's deaths were children under the age of one, reflective of a profound lack of progress on water quality and infant mortality.[150]

PUBLIC HEALTH AND EPIDEMIOLOGIC TRANSITIONS

Public health campaigns hastened Yucatán's epidemiologic transition. Abdel Omran's concept of "epidemiologic transitions" envisions three stages, though others have added a fourth. Mortality rates are quite high during the first stage, primarily due to epidemic disease and famine. Mortality rates begin to fall in the second stages, as epidemic disease and famine become less frequent, though infectious diseases remain the leading cause of death. Omran's third stage sees the control of most infectious disease, a decline in rates of infant mortality and the emergence of endemic diseases as the leading causes of death. "Man-made" causes of death, associated with lifestyle, socioeconomic factors, diet, and the like become increasingly common in the third stage. A final stage has been proposed, with continued low mortality rates, but increased rates of nonlethal diseases that compromise the quality of life.[151] These transitions are clear in changing mortality rates in the region. (This topic is discussed in chapter 6.)

Though officials in 1910 might know that tuberculosis and water quality were leading causes of death, institutional capacity, technological ability, and social mission limited the diseases they chose to attack. The focus of public health campaigns was upon epidemic diseases such as smallpox and yellow fever. The *Junta Superior de Sanidad* directed little of its institutional energies against the most common causes of death in the region. The control of these "crowd killer" diseases accentuated the presence of contagious diseases and paid less attention to those associated with water quality and living conditions.

Although physicians associated with the *Sociedad Médica Yucateca* played crucial roles in the campaigns against contagious diseases, not all were happy with the public health agenda. Rafael Betancourt criticized the limited social agenda of public health in the region at a 1911 meeting of the Yucatec Medical Society. While the Society had proven to be an excellent source of solidarity and knowledge of new medical ideas, it had failed in its social mission. Betancourt cited the roles of younger physicians in Europe who were tackling issues such as lowering infant mortality. Yucatán had some of the higher rates in Latin America. Cuba and Uruguay had lowered their rates—why couldn't Yucatán? The body needed to form a commission to approach the governor,[152] a proposal that yielded no response from a regime more concerned with falling henequen prices than the reduction of infant mortality.

A partnership among the medical corps, governmental agencies, and society would be required to combat infant mortality in Betancourt's opinion. Drawing upon both international and domestic precedents, Germán Pompeyo offered a series of eugenic actions intended to reduce the region's infant mortality rate. A first step would be to increase the age of legal marriage from the current levels of 14 for females and 16 for males. Young people of this age, Pompeyo asserted, were not physically mature and could not produce "robust and healthy" babies, leading to the "degeneration of the race." Agencies of the state government should enforce the educational dimensions of the Sanitary Codes that would enable schools to teach hygiene to the "mothers of tomorrow." More innovative would be the creation of "Healthy Infant Brigades" modeled after efforts taken in the United States. These brigades would consist of professional women who would undertake a campaign of public education, including the distribution of pamphlets and the sponsorship of conferences. One goal of the Healthy Infant Brigades would be to create

"Leagues of Mothers," young women who would teach others on how to "save the child." Finally, Pompeyo called for a Professional Association to review and propose public health laws that the Brigades would use in their statewide effort.[153] José C. Villamil, a resident of Tekax, suggested that the School of Medicine create a two-year course that would instill basic septic and nutritional concepts among the state's midwives.[154]

Prenatal training and social programs could also stem the malnutrition that plagued Yucatán's rural children. The Carnegie Report, conducted in the early 1930s, demonstrated many medical deficiencies in rural communities. Commenting on the report, Alvar Carrillo Gil stated that 75 percent of rural population suffered severe dietary problems. Improved dietary habits, such as the consumption of more protien, vegetables, and platanos would reduce the chronic malnutrition.[155]

This limited social agenda yielded little concerted activity by public health officials to affect the quotidian health conditions in Yucatán. Advocates of social medicine had little influence upon the actions of the region's public health system. Diseases more firmly rooted in socioeconomic structures were addressed in the interior only with the construction of a public health infrastructure in the 1930s and 1940s. With public health agencies lacking a dynamic social mission, residents suffered from diseases that could have been addressed by officials with a distinct mindset.

NOTES

1. Joseph White to Wickliffe Rose, August 4, 1914, Record Group (RG) 5.1.1 (pre-1915), Box 11, Folder 177. Rockefeller Foundation Archives, Rockefeller Archive Center, Sleepy Hollow, New York (hereafter designated RAC).

2. Joaquín Patrón and Agustín Cáceres M. to Lazaro J. Barrera, January 7, 13, 1903, Mérida, AGEY, FPE, Sección JSS, Serie Copiador de Oficios, Vol. 11, entries 5816, 5817, 5818, 5831.

3. Patrón and Cáceres to Yuanuario Manzanilla, May 12, 1903, Mérida, AGEY, FPE, Sección JSS, Serie Copiador de Oficios, Vol. 11, entry 6371; ibid. to Governor, May 16, 1903, ibid., 6381.

4. Patrón and Císares to Governor, August 21, 1903, September 15, 1903, December 10, 1903, Mérida, AGEY, FPE, Sección JSS, Serie Copiador de Oficios, Vol. 12, entries 6908, 7042, 7360. See also Harald Seidelin, "Report of Yellow Fever Expedition to Yucatán, 1911–1912," *Yellow Fever Bureau Bulletin* 2:2 (October 1912), 152–53.

5. Alfred W. Crosby Jr., *The Columbian Exchange: Biological and Cultural Consequences of 1492* (Westport, CT: Greenwood Press, 1972), 46.

6. F. Fenner, D. A. Henderson, I. Arita, Z. Ježek, I. D. Ladnyi, *Smallpox and its Eradication* (Geneva: World Health Organization, 1988), 236.

7. "Measles," Center for Disease Control, http://www2.ncid.cdc.gov/travel/yb/utils/ybGet.asp?section=dis&obj=measles.htm (accessed, May 14, 2006).

8. David Noble Cook, *Born to Die: Disease and New World Conquest, 1492–1650* (Cambridge: Cambridge University Press, 1998), 86–91.

9. "Plague," Center for Disease Control, http://www.cdc.gov/ncidod/dvbid/plague/epi.htm (Accessed, May 14, 2006).

10. Crosby, *The Columbian Exchange*, 97.

11. Cook, *Born to Die*, 89–90, 108–09, 115–16.

12. John M. Barry, *The Great Influenza: The Epic Story of the Deadliest Plague in History* (New York: Penguin Books, 2004).

13. Cook, *Born to Die*, 32–33, 53–56, 86.

14. Roy Porter, *The Greatest Benefit to Mankind: A Medical History of Humanity* (New York: W. W. Norton, 1997), 20–22.

15. Cook, *Born to Die*, 49–50; J. N. Hays, *The Burdens of Disease Epidemics and Human Response in Western History* (New Brunswick, N.J.: Rutgers University Press, 1998), 74, 207.

16. Sherburne F. Cook and Woodrow Borah, "The Population of Yucatán, 1517–1960," in *Essays in Population History: Mexico and the Caribbean*, 3 vols. (Berkeley: University of California Press, 1974), Vol. 2, 114–20.

17. Farriss, *Maya Society under Colonial Rule*, 74–76, 201–02.

18. Kenneth F. Kiple and Brian T. Higgins, "Yellow Fever and the Africanization of the Caribbean," in *Disease and Demography in the Americas*, ed. by John W. Verano and Douglas H. Ubelaker (Washington: Smithsonian Institution Press, 1992), 238–41.

19. Henry Rose Carter claimed that this was the first direct observation of the disease in the Americas, but that it clearly originated in Africa. *Yellow Fever: An Epidemiological and Historical Study of its Place of Origin* (Baltimore: The Williams & Wilkins Company, 1931), 265, 270–71. Miguel E. Bustamante asserts that an outbreak of "xekik" in 1464 was urban yellow fever. *La fiebre amarilla en México y su origen en America* (México DF: Instituto de Salubridad y Enfermedades Tropicales de la Secretaría de Salubridad y Asistencia, 1958), 5.

20. López de Cogollado, as cited by Farriss, *Maya Society under Colonial Rule*, 84; Robert Patch, *Maya and Spaniard in Yucatán, 1648–1812* (Stanford: Stanford University Press, 1993), 42–44.

21. Cook and Borah, "Population of Yucatán," 114, 122–23.

22. Fenner, *Smallpox and Its Eradication*, 245–57.

23. Catherine Mark and José G. Rigau-Pérez, "The World's First Immunization Campaign: The Spanish Smallpox Vaccine Expedition, 1803–1813," *Bulletin of the History of Medicine* 83:1 (Spring 2009), 63–94; Arturo Erosa Barbachano, *La Escuela de Medicina de Mérida, Yucatán* (Mérida: Ediciones de la Universidad Autónoma de Yucatán, 1997), 23.

24. *La Emulación*, January 1875.

25. McCrea, *Diseased Relations*, chapter 2.

26. McCrea, *Diseased Relations*, 33.

27. Seidelin, "Yellow Fever Expedition," 155.

28. Charles E. Rosenberg, *The Cholera Years: The United States in 1832, 1849, and 1866* (Chicago: University of Chicago Press, 1987).
29. Erosa Barbachano, *La Escuela de Medicina de* Mérida, 34–35.
30. *La Emulación*, November 1874.
31. *La Emulación*, January 1875.
32. *La Emulación*, June 1875.
33. *Boletín de Higiene*, September 10, 1895.
34. *La Emulación*, February 1875.
35. *La Emulación*, June, 1874, August 1876, January 1879. See McCrea, *Diseased Relations*, chapter three, for a discussion of nineteenth-century burial history.
36. *La Emulación*, January 1879.
37. Marcus Cueto, *The Value of Heath: A History of the Pan American Health Organization* (Washington, DC: Pan American Health Organization, 2007), 11–13.
38. Douglas M. Haynes, *Imperial Medicine: Patrick Manson and the Conquest of Tropical Disease* (Philadelphia: University of Pennsylvania Press, 2001), 36–41.
39. Helen J. Power, *Tropical Medicine in the Twentieth Century: A History of Liverpool School of Tropical Medicine* (London: Kegan Paul International, 1999), 13–14; Michael Worbys, "Manson, Ross and colonial medical policy: tropical medicine in London and Liverpool, 1899–1914," in *Disease, Medicine, and Empire: Perspectives on Western Medicine and the Experience of European Expansion*, ed. by Roy Macleod and Milton Lewis (New York: Routledge, 1988), 21–37.
40. Carlos E. Finlay, *Carlos Finlay and Yellow Fever* (New York: The Institute of Tropical Medicine of the University of Havana, Oxford University Press, 1940), 50–54, 58–75; Carter, *Yellow Fever*; Mariola Espinosa, *Epidemic Invasions: Yellow Fever and the Limits of Cuban Independence, 1878–1930* (Chicago: Chicago University Press, 2009), 55–66; Molly Caldwell Crosby, *The American Plague: The Untold Story of Yellow Fever. The Epidemic that Shaped our History* (New York: Berkley Books, 2006), 203–04; François Delaporte, trans. by Arthur Goldhammer, *The History of Yellow Fever: An Essay on the Birth of Tropical Medicine* (Cambridge: The MIT Press, 1991) suggests Finlay's unrecognized debt to Patrick Manson, 33–63.
41. Cueto, *The Value of Heath*, 39–44, 48–49; Carlos Viesca Treviño, "Eduardo Liceaga y la Participación Mexicana en la Fundación de la Organización Panamericana de la Salud," *Revista Cubana de Salud Pública* 24:1 (1998), 11–18.
42. Ralph Chester Williams, *The United States Public Health Service, 1798–1950* (Washington DC: Commissioned Officers Association of the United States Public Health Service, 1951), 446–47; Cueto, *The Value of Heath*, 63–65.
43. McCrea, *Diseased Relations*, 54–56.
44. JSS to jefe político del partido de Ticul, Mérida, July 14, 1891, AGEY, FPE, Sec. JSS, Copiador de Oficios, Vol. 1, entry 40.
45. Correspondence concerning vaccinations dominate *Junta Superior de Sanidad* records in the 1890s.
46. *Boletín de Higiene*, May 25, 1895.
47. *Boletín de Higiene*, October 10, December 10, 1895.
48. Joaquín Patrón and Agustín Caceres to Jefe Político de Mérida, December 8, 1902, Mérida, AGEY, FPE, Sec. JSS, Serie Copiador de Oficios, Vol. 11, entry 5719.

49. Patrón to Cáceres M. to Governor, January 23, 1903, Mérida, AGEY, FPE, Sección JSS, Serie Copiador de Oficios, Volume 11, entry 5881.

50. McCrea, *Diseased Relations*, footnote, 218–19.

51. *Boletín de Higiene*, September 10, 1895.

52. *Boletin de Sanitario*, April 11, 21, 22, 1908.

53. Gustavo Vega and Rojas Aguilar to governor, March 23, 1908, AGEY, FPE, Sec. JSS, Serie Copiador de Oficios, Volume 17, entry, 73.

54. *La Higiene*, June 1918.

55. The development of the disease and the public health response to it can be traced in AGEY, FPE, Sec. Beneficencia, Serie Sanidad, 1915, Caja 479.

56. JSS to Governor, August 6, 1915, Mérida, AGEY, FPE, Sec. Beneficencia Pública, Serie Sanidad, 1915, Caja 478.

57. *La Higiene*, June 1918.

58. Alvaro Torre Díaz, *Cuatro años en el Gobierno de Yucatán, 1926–1930* (Mérida: Compañía Tipográfica Yucateca, 1930), 99.

59. José Ronzón, *Sanidad y modernización en los puertos del Alto Caribe,* 1870–1915 (México DF: Universidad Autónoma Metropolitana, 2004), 9.

60. Cueto, *The Value of Heath*, 25.

61. *Boletín de Higiene*, May 25, 1895.

62. Patrón and Césares M. to Governor, August 21, September 15, December 10, 1903, Mérida, AGEY, FPE, Sec. JSS, Serie Copiador de Oficios, Vol. 12, entries 6908, 7042, 7360.

63. Ana María Carrilllo, "Guerra de exterminio al 'Fantasma de las costas': La primera campaña contra la fiebre amarilla en México, 1903–1911," in *Curar, Sanar y Educar: Enfermedad y Sociedad en México Siglos XIX y XX*, Coord. by Claudia Agostoni (México DF: Universidad Nacional Autónoma de México; Benemérita Universidad Autónoma de Puebla, 2008), 223, 226, 229–30, 238; Fernando Martínez Cortés and Xochitl Martínez Barbosa, *El Consejo Superior de Salubridad: Rector de la Salud Pública en* México (México DF: SmithKline Beecham Mexico, 1997), 156.

64. Eduardo Liceaga (Jefe Consejo Superior de Salubridad) to Secretario de Gobernación, México, August 27, 1906, ASSHA, Fondo de Salubridad Pública (FSP), Sec. Salubridad en Territorios, Puertos y Fronteras, Caja 2, Exp. 5; E. Ruiz to Secretario de Gobernación, August 17, 1906, AHSSA, FSP, Sec. Salubridad en Territorios, Puertos y Fronteras, Caja 2, Expediente 5; Carrilllo, "Guerra de exterminio," 223, 226, 229–30, 238.

65. Typical of the order to cover cisterns was Joaquín Patrón and Agustín Cáceres to Artaldo Erosa, May 19, 1908, Mérida, AGEY, FPE, Sec. JSS, Serie Copiador de Oficios, Volume17, entry 383. See also entries, 384–94. On the 1904 order, see Patrón and Cáceres to Delegado de Consejo Superior de Sanidad, June 26, 1908, Mérida, AGEY, FPE, Sec. JSS, Serie Copiador de Oficios, Vol. 18, entry 43.

66. See, for example, Patrón and Cáceres to Delegado de Consejo Superior de Sanidad, October 21, 1908, Mérida, AGEY, FPE, Sec. JSS, Serie Copiador de Oficios, Volume 19, entry 16.

67. *La Revista Médica de Yucatán*, February 1906.

68. *La Revista Médica de Yucatán*, December 1912.

69. Bustamante, *La fiebre amarilla en México*, 118.

70. Expedición de la Escuela de Medicina Tropical de Liverpool, 1911–1912, *Informe de la expedición para investigar la fiebre amarilla en Yucatán, por el Dr. HARALD SEIDELIN* (Mérida: Imprenta "el Porvenir," 1914), 5.

71. Alejandro Cevera-Andrade, "Harald Seidelin. Su labor in Yucatán, México," *Revista Biomédica* 17:3 (July-September 2002), 223.

72. Seidelin, "Yellow Fever Expedition," 124, 201–05.

73. Rafael Betancourt Agramonte, *Remitente Biliosa forma hemorrágica de a corre en los nativos de Yucatán* (Mérida: Tip. y Lit. "La Moderna," 1913), 7–9; Seidelin, "Yellow Fever expedition," 125, 127–32.

74. Seidelin, "Yellow Fever expedition," 203–09.

75. The most detailed studies are Armando Solorzano, "The Rockefeller Foundation in Revolutionary Mexico: Yellow Fever in Yucatán and Veracruz," in Marcos Cueto, ed., *Missionaries of Science: The Rockefeller Foundation and Latin America* (Bloomington: Indiana University Press, 1994), 52–71, and McCrea, *Diseased Relations*, 171–89. See also Alexandra Minna Stern, "Yellow Fever Crusade: US Colonialism, Tropical Medicine, and the International Politics of Mosquito Control, 1900–1920," in *Disease, Globalization and Security, 1850 to the Present*, ed. by Alison Bashford (London: Palgrave MacMillan, 2006), 41–59; Anne-Emanuelle Birn, *Marriage of Convenience: Rockefeller International Health and Revolutionary Mexico* (Rochester NY: University of Rochester Press, 2006); Dr. Pedro Cámara-Milán, "El Dr. Hideyo Noguchi en Yucatán," *Revista Biomédica* 11 (2000), 207–212; Ilana Löwy, "Epidemiology, Immunology, and Yellow Fever: The Rockefeller Foundation in Brazil, 1923–1939," *Journal of the History of Biology* 30 (1997), 397–417; Steven Palmer, *Launching Global Health: The Caribbean Odyssey of the Rockefeller Foundation* (Ann Arbor: The University of Michigan Press, 2010); Farley, *To Cast Out Disease*, 37–39. For an analysis of the hookworm campaign in Costa Rica, see Palmer, *From Popular Medicine to Medical Populism,* 155–82; for Mexico, see Anne-Emanuelle Birn, "Revolution, the Scatological Way: The Rockefeller Foundation's Hookworm Campaign in 1920s Mexico," in *Disease in the History of Modern Latin America: From Malaria to AIDS*, ed. by Diego Armus (Durham: Duke University Press, 2003), 158–82.

76. Isabel R. Plesset, *Noguchi and His Patrons* (Rutherford, NJ: Fairleigh Dickinson University Press, 1980), 176–91; Marcos Cueto, "The cycles of eradication: the Rockefeller Foundation and Latin American Public Health," in *International health organisations and movements,* 1918–1939, Ed. by Paul Weindling (Cambridge: Cambridge University Press, 1995), 229; Paul Franklin Clark, "Hideyo Noguchi, 1876–1928," *Bulletin of the History of Medicine* 33: No. 1 (January–February 1959), 17–18; Elmer Bendiner, "Noguchi: Many Triumphs and a Brilliant Failure," *Hospital Practice* 19:2 (February 1984), 247–54; George W. Corner, *A History of the Rockefeller Institute,* 1901–1953*: Origins and Growth* (New York: The Rockefeller Institute Press, 1964), 190.

77. *La Revista Médica de Yucatán*, January 1920.

78. *La Revista Médica de Yucatán*, January 1920.

79. Plesset, *Noguchi and His Patrons*, 192–204.

80. Gil Rojas to Alfonso Pruneda, Mérida, March 30, 1921, ASSHA, FSP, Sec. Epidemiología, Caja 17, Exp. 3; "Memoria de la Segunda Convención de Fiebre Amarilla, Agosto 1–3 de 1922," ASSHA, FSP, Sec. Congresos y Convenciones, Caja 12, Exp. 8.

81. Gil Rojas to Junta Superior de Sanidad, October 25, 1920, Mérida, AGEY, FPE, Sec. Beneficencia, Caja 717.

82. Clark, "Hideyo Noguchi," 18–19.

83. Connor, "Notes on Yellow Fever in Mexico," October 15, 1923, Mérida, RAC, RG 5.2 (IHB Special Reports), Box 33, Series 323, Folder 193; Connor, "Final Report. Yellow Fever, Merida, Yucatán, Mexico," RAC, RG 5, Series 323, Box 33, folder 194, 1–3.

84. Rojas Aguilar to Departamento de Salubridad Pública, Mérida, November 30, 1922, ASSHA, FSP, Sec. Epidemiología, Caja 21, Exp. 17; Rojas Aguilar to Alfonso Pruneda, Mérida, March 30, 1921, ASSHA, FSP, Sec. Epidemiología, Caja 17, Exp. 3.

85. Diego Hernández F. to Roberto Medellín, Jefe DSP, Mérida, December 20, 1924, ASSHA, FSP, Sec. Salubridad en Territorios, Puertos y Fronteras, Caja 3, Exp. 12.

86. C. E. Athey to Public Health and Marine Hospital Service, April 1, 1926, Mérida, United States National Archive and Record Administration (NARA), RG 90, Records of the Public Health Service, General Subject File, 1924–35, Foreign Stations Immigration, Progres[o] (Mexico), Box 790, 0960–136.

87. Birn, *Marriage of Convenience*, 58–59.

88. "Memoria de la Segunda Convención de Fiebre Amarilla, Agosto 1–3 de 1922," ASSHA, FSP, Sec. Congresos y Convenciones, Caja 12, Exp. 8.

89. Pedro F. Rivas, "Prophylaxis of Yellow Fever in Yucatán," RAC, RG 2 (stack material), series 323 (1927), Box 551, folder 3680, 5–6, 7, 10.

90. Carrillo, "Guerra de exterminio," 248–49.

91. Diego Hernández F. to Roberto Medellín, Jefe DSP, Mérida, December 20, 1924, ASSHA, FSP, Sec. Salubridad en Territorios, Puertos y Fronteras, Caja 3, Exp. 12.

92. Athey to the Public Health and Marine Hospital Service, April 1, 1926, NARA, RG 90, Records of the Public Health Service General Subject File, 1924–1935. Foreign Stations Immigration. Progress, Mexico. Box 790.

93. For a readable account of efforts to cure malaria, see Mark Honigsbaum, *The Fever Trail: In Search of the Cure for Malaria* (New York: Farrar, Straus and Giroux, 2001).

94. Shattuck, *The Peninsula of Yucatán*, 358.

95. JSS to Governor, January 17, 1922, Mérida, AGEY, FPE, Sec. Beneficencia y Sanidad, Serie Correspondencia (Sanidad), año 1922, Caja 753 bis.

96. Municipal Council President to Governor, February 18, 1922, Hocabá; Governor to Hocobá Municipal Council President, February 24, 1922, Mérida, AGEY, FPE, Sec. Beneficencia y Sanidad, Serie Correspondencia (Sanidad), año 1922, Caja 753 bis.

97. Shattuck, *The Peninsula of Yucatán*, 360.

98. *La Revista Médica de Yucatán* (October 1934).

99. Departamento de Salubridad Pública, *Informe general del Departamento de Salubridad que comprende las labores a cabo durante la administración de C. Lic.*

Emilio Portes Gil, siendo Jefe del Departamento el C. Dr. Aquilino Villanueva (Mexico: Talleres del Imp. del Departamento de Salubridad Pública, 1930), 48–49.

100. *Informe del Ciudadano Professor José González Beytia Gobernador Constitucional del Estado, año de 1949* (Mérida: Talleres Gráficos Edit. Zamná, 1949), 113.

101. Marcos Cueto, *Cold War, Deadly Fevers: Malaria Eradication in Mexico, 1955–1975* (Washington DC: Woodrow Wilson Center Press, The Johns Hopkins University Press, 2007).

102. *La Higiene*, February 1919, 338.

103. Gil Rojas to Governor, January 24 and 28, 1919, Mérida, AGEY, FPE, Sección JSS, Serie Copiador de Oficios, Volume 81, entries 103, 137.

104. Gil Rojas to Governor, February 3, 1919, Mérida, AGEY, FPE, Serie Beneficencia Sanidad y Salubridad, Caja 679.

105. *La Higiene*, February 1919.

106. *La Higiene*, March 1919.

107. *La Higiene*, June 1919.

108. Smith, *Gender and the Mexican Revolution*, 148.

109. Jorge I. Castillo Canché and José E. Serrano Catzín, "Vigilar y normal el burdel: legalización de la prostitución femenina en Yucatán durante el porfiriato," *Revista de la Universidad Autónoma de Yucatán* No. 188 (January/February/March 1994), 47–48.

110. *Código sanitario del Estado de Yucatán* (Mérida: Imprenta de la "Escuela Correccional del Artes y Oficios," 1911), 70–71.

111. Castillo Canché and Serrano Catzín, "Vigilar y normal el burdel," 50–51, 54.

112. Patrón and Cásares to Governor, September 29, 1903, Mérida, AGEY, FPE, Sec. JSS, Serie Copiador de Oficios, Volume 12, entry 7082.

113. Jefe de la JSS to Jefe Político, Mérida, December 19, 1909, Mérida, AGEY, FPE, sec. JSS, Serie Copiador de Oficios, Volume 18, entry 50.

114. "Al Gobernado del Estado," Mérida, October 10, 1908, AGEY, FPE, Sec. Beneficencia, Series Hospitales, Sanidad, Correspondencia, old Caja 275, new caja 592.

115. Gustavo Vega to the Jefe Político de Mérida, January 6, 1914, Mérida, AGEY, FPE, Sec. JSS, Serie Copiador de Oficios, Vol. 54, entry 55.

116. W. G. Cantón to Jefe Político de Mérida, June 21, 1899, Mérida, AGEY, FPE, Sec. JSS, Serie Copiador de Oficios, Volume 6, entry 1445.

117. Joaguín Patrón to Cásares, December 8, 1902, Mérida, AGEY, FPE, Sección JSS, Serie Copiador de Oficios, Volume 11, entry 5719.

118. *La Higiene*, March 1919.

119. JSS to Governor, January 17, 1922, Mérida, AGEY, FPE, Sección Beneficencia y Sanidad, Serie Correspondencia (Sanidad), año 1922, Caja 753 bis.

120. *Informe rendido al gobernador constitucional de Yucatán c. Dr. Alvaro Torre Díaz, ante la XXX Legislatura del Estado el 1° de Enero de 1928* (Mérida: Talleres Tipográficos del Gobierno del Estado, 1928), 14.

121. Donna J. Guy, "Medical Imperialism Gone Awry: The Campaign Against Legalized Prostitution in Latin America," in Meade and Walker, editors. *Science, Medicine and Cultural Imperialism* (New York: St. Martin's Press, 1991), 75–94.

122. *La Emulación*, February 1878.

123. *La Emulación*, February 1878.

124. JSS to Governor, May 29, 1922, Mérida, AGEY, FPE, Sección Beneficencia y Sanidad, Serie Correspondencia (Sanidad), año 1922, Caja 753 bis.

125. *La Higiene*, June 1918.

126. *La Higiene*, May 1918.

127. Torre Díaz, *Cuatro años en el Gobierno de Yucatán,*, 98.

128. José María Salazar A. to Governor, March 5, 1934, Mérida, AGEY, FPE, Sección JSS, Serie Copiador de Oficios, Volume 161, entry 606.

129. *Informe del Ciudadano Professor José González Beytia*, 72–73.

130. Diego Armus, *The Ailing City: Health, Tuberculosis, and Culture in Buenos Aires, 1870–1950* (Durham: Duke University Press, 2011).

131. Porter, *The Greatest Benefit to Mankind,* 309–12, 437, 457–58, 693–94.

132. *La Revista Médica de Yucatán*, December 1905.

133. *La Revista Médica de Yucatán*, February 1910.

134. Shattuck, *The Peninsula of Yucatán*, 366.

135. Eduardo Aguilar Gómez "El problema de la lucha anti-tuberculosa en Yucatán: Base para abordarlo," in Congreso Médico Peninsular, *Memorias del segundo congreso médico peninsular* (Mérida: Díaz Massa, 1945), 281.

136. Departamento de Salubridad Pública, *Informe general*, 13–14; Aguilar Gómez, "La lucha anti-tuberculosa," 280–82.

137. "Informe extenso de las labores desarrolladas por la Oficina de la Campaña contra la Tuberculosis, del 1° de Septiembre de 1941 al 31 de Agosto del presente año [1942]," Mérida, July 31, 1942, AHSSA, FSP, Sección Presidencia, Serie Secretaria, Caja 15, Exp. 3.

138. José F. Diaz and Benjamín Gongora Triay, "La higiene," in *Enciclopedia Yucatenense* (México DF: Edición Oficial del Gobierno de Yucatán, 1977), vol. VI, 420.

139. Aguilar Gómez "El problema de la lucha anti-tuberculosa," 285.

140. *Asistencia Social* 1:2 (October, November, December 1948), 42–43.

141. Shattuck, *The Peninsula of Yucatán*, 362.

142. Wells and Joseph, "Chilango Modernization," 195. For the Mexico City "model" followed by Yucatec modernizers, see Claudia Agostini, *Monuments of Progress: Modernization and Public Health in Mexico City, 1876–1910* (Calgary: University of Calgary Press, 2003).

143. Memorandum on the "Chemical Analysis of water in Mérida," in Hernan C. Vogentiz, American Vice-Counsel, to the Department of State, Mérida, November 3, 1924, Records of the Public Health Service, General Subject File, 1924–1936, NARA, RG 90, Box 830, folder 4, 6.

144. "Chemical Analysis of water in Mérida," Records of the Public Health Service, General Subject File, 1924–1936, NARA, RG 90, Box 830, folder 4, 9.

145. *La Revista Médica de Yucatán*, April 1943.

146. Shattuck, *The Peninsula of Yucatán*, 363.

147. *La Revista Médica de Yucatán*, August 1946.

148. *La Revista Médica de Yucatán*, September 1911.

149. *La Revista Médica de Yucatán*, December 1923.

150. *La Revista Médica de Yucatán*, April 1943.

151. Abdel R. Omran, "The Epidemiological Transition Theory: A Theory of the Epidemiology of Population Change," *Milbank Memorial Fund Quarterly* 49 (1971), 509–38; Rosario Cárdenas, "Las causas de muerte en México," in *La población de México: Tendencias y perspectivas sociodemográficas hacia el siglo XXI*, coordinated by José Gómez de León Cruces and Cecilia Rabell Romero (México DF: Consejo Nacional de Población, Fondo de Cultura Económica, 2001), 117.

152. *La Revista Médica de Yucatán*, September 1911.

153. Copy of a speech made in January 1922, published in *La Revista Médica de Yucatán,* December 1924.

154. *La Revista Médica de Yucatán,* February 1936.

155. *La Revista Médica de Yucatán*, June 1935.

Chapter 5

Public Health and the Revolutionary State

Yucatec public health officials frustrated Pedro Castillo Cervera, the Federal Sanitary Delegate at the port of Progreso. The Mexican constitution of 1857 and the new revolutionary charter of 1917 had given the federal government explicit jurisdiction over communicable diseases and public health in the nation's ports. The *Junta Superior de Sanidad* in Mérida, however, insisted that all ships leaving the port present proof of smallpox inoculations to *Junta* officials under the express authorization of Governor Carrillo Puerto. Failure to do so would violate state statutes and warrant a hefty fine. Castillo Cervera appealed to his superior, Dr. Alfonso Pruneda, the secretary general of the *Departamento de Salubridad Pública*, seeking the assertion of federal authority. Appropriately, Pruneda rejected the Yucatec governor's assertion, informing Castillo Cervera that the port fell under federal jurisdiction, not that of Yucatán. To Prudena, this was part of a Yucatec pattern of such "incursions" on federal authority.[1]

This seemingly minor incident suggests the tensions between the state and federal governments in the arena of public health. Sanitary delegations constituted the primary federal health presence in Yucatán, delegations that often raised questions of jurisdictional authority.[2] Yucatán, after all, had developed its own public health system and its elite skillfully protected their positions of power and sense of regional autonomy. While the regime of Porfirio Díaz subordinated the Yucatec periphery to the political and military authority of central Mexico, wealth from henequen production enabled Yucatán to construct a public health system reflective of its own priorities. The Revolution, however, expanded the rights and powers of federal public health officials. In the 1920s, DSP officials sought the expansion of Mexican state authority over Yucatec officials in keeping with their new vision of the Mexican state.

Even the ardent revolutionary Carrillo Puerto would resist the expansion of federal authority over Yucatec operations.

By the 1930s, political stability, revolutionary vision, and institutional capacity greatly expanded the reach of the Mexican state. This enabled the Cárdenas presidency to undertake an ambitious effort to bring health care to thousands of rural residents. The land reforms of Cárdenas included the confiscation of Yucatec henequen estates and the mandate that *ejidos* have access to "modern" health care. President Manuel Ávila Camacho (1940–1946) fulfilled the promise of the Constitution of 1917 by the creation of the Secretary of Health and Assistance (*Secretaría de Salubridad y Asistencia*, SSA) and the Mexican Institute of Social Security (*Instituto Mexicano del Seguro Social*, IMSS), organizations that promised "modern" health care to all Mexicans. These public health initiatives, along with similar educational measures, situated the state in the daily lives of most Mexicans.

Public health initiatives made biomedicine a part of the daily life of Yucatec residents, an "everyday form of state formation" advanced by both the Mexican and Yucatec governments. Residents learned habits of "good health" through public health activities, just as they learned how to be citizens through the school system. As Elise Rockwell points out, the state formation process was by no means coherent, nor was it an uncontested "top-down" process.[3] In Yucatán, two governmental bodies, one Yucatec and one Mexican, engaged in a protracted struggle for control of the region's public health infrastructure. Revolutionary state formation required a Mexican victory. Given the largely autonomous development of the public health system in Yucatán, how did revolutionary health policies affect this historic relationship? The role of public health in Mexican state formation in Yucatán is the central theme of this chapter.[4]

THE FEDERAL PUBLIC HEALTH SYSTEM

Colonial institutions slowly gave way to a modern public health infrastructure over the course of the nineteenth century in Mexico City. President Anastacio Bustamante (1830–1832) suppressed the *protomedicato* in 1831, transferring its authority to the newly created Medical Faculty of the Federal District (*Facultad Médica del Distrito Federal*). (In time, this would become the Faculty of Medicine of the National Autonomous University of Mexico—UNAM.) The *Consejo Superior de Salubridad* (Supreme Health Board), created in 1841, lasted until the Revolution, when it was replaced by the *Departamento de Salubridad Pública*. The medical school continued as an autonomous and collaborative institution with the *Consejo Superior*. Most of the functions of the *Consejo Superior* came directly from the *protomedicato*, including guiding oversight of the practice of medicine, the right to issue and register titles, monitoring of pharmacies, and preserving for titled physicians, surgeons, dentists, bleeders, and midwives the legal authority to practice medicine. It had public health functions, notably the preparation of smallpox vaccine.[5]

Dr. Eduardo Liceaga oversaw the modernization of the public health system of the federal government.[6] Liceaga served as director of the *Consejo Superior* from 1885 until 1914, a time of momentous changes in the activities of the body. Liceaga used his personal friendship with President Díaz to expand the powers of the office, developing modern laboratory facilities, attending to Mexico City's sanitation system, and regularizing vaccination programs. His leadership led to passage of a new federal sanitary code in 1891 and a significant growth in the number of public health employees. By the end of the century, the *Consejo Superior* operated some twenty-four vaccination stations in Mexico City, employed thousands, and was present at most points of entry into the country.[7]

The 1891 Federal Sanitary Code did not alter the fundamental constraints on federal authority, but it did introduce modern, sanitarian approaches to disease. The government expressed concern about contagious diseases, perhaps because they might threaten the economic boom of the Porfiriato. Federal authority was thus extended to ports and points of entry, making the *Consejo Superior* responsible for blocking epidemic diseases, unhealthy drugs, and bad food from entering the country. It also empowered the government to work with states on questions of hygiene and public health, though always at the invitation of local authorities. Federal delegations monitored the ports of Campeche and Vera Cruz, as well as Progreso, Sisal, and Celestún, the first sustained federal health presence in Yucatán.[8] These agents were primarily concerned with the control of diseases that could damage the trading networks of the upper Caribbean.

The *Consejo Superior* aggressively expanded its public health campaigns. In 1902, for example, the plague entered Mexico through trade relations with San Francisco. Federal authorities dispatched agents to Mazatlán, significantly reducing its impact. In describing the federal response to this epidemic, Ana María Carrillo outlines other campaigns against syphilis, malaria, smallpox, tuberculosis, and, most extensively, yellow fever.[9]

The 1903 campaign against yellow fever symbolized Liceaga's expansion of federal public health concerns. Convinced by the success of the US program against yellow fever in Havana, Liceaga engineered a nationwide campaign against the disease after an outbreak in Veracruz. Yucatec officials at first declined to cooperate with the federal delegates. The governor insisted that the federal government had no right to intrude upon the state's jurisdiction, and that the state could not be forced to finance the operation.[10]

Reconciliation soon permitted federal agents to assume a lead role in the anti-yellow fever campaign, which included the visitation of hotels, oiling of standing waters, the dispensation of quinine pills, and monitoring open water containers.[11] Disputes over funding the program, however, persisted.

The Mexican Revolution dramatically reduced the scope of the *Consejo Superior*. It drew back to the Mexico City region, leaving unchallenged the diseases and social trauma of the war in most of the nation. Mexican yellow fellow delegates withdrew from Yucatán in the early days of the Revolution, leaving local physician Gil Rojas Aguilar as the Federal Sanitary Delegate in Mérida.[12] Gustavo Vega, head of the JSS, worked closely with the federal sanitary delegation in Progreso, developing plans to close the port in the face of disease threats in the upper Caribbean trade network.[13] As José María Rodríguez replaced Liceaga as head of the *Consejo Superior* in 1914, he took charge of a system that had improved conditions for many elite and middle class Mexicans, but, in Anne-Emanuelle Birn's assertion, had left "most of the population [living] under public health conditions comparable to those they had endured through the colonial period."[14]

REVOLUTION *DESDE AFUERA*—1910s AND 1920s

The Revolution came to Yucatán from the outside and sputtered through several periods of ineffective reformist activity. Colonel Abel Ortiz Argumedo seized control of the state government in February 1915, supported by the henequen and political elite who sought to preempt more a radical Constitutionalist intervention. General Venustiano Carranza proved unhappy with the rapprochement; an army under General Salvador Alvarado occupied Mérida on March 19.[15]

Alvarado proved to be an ambitious reformer. A wave of decrees ended debt peonage, reorganized municipal governments, and founded scores of schools and libraries. Alvarado helped to establish peasant and workers' *Ligas de Resistencia* (Resistance Leagues) as a base of power for the newly created *Partido Socialista de Yucatán*. He severed relations between Molina Solís and International Harvester and founded a state agency to manage henequen sales—and to siphon money in support the war effort. Alvarado generated considerable elite opposition by his antipathy toward the Church, efforts to mobilize workers, and zeal to limit public "vice." That, in combination with falling henequen prices, would curtail many of the reforms and lead to his recall to Mexico City in 1918.[16]

With Alvarado came a revolutionary vision for Yucatec health care. Alvarado insisted that it was the responsibility of the government to assist the poor, especially during periods of economic unrest. In August of 1915, he decreed the creation of free clinics in five of Mérida's poorest neighborhoods. Each barrio would have a full-time physician and a pharmacist. Consultations would be free, but visitors would have to pay twenty percent of the cost of each prescription. The governor's office would pay for these services,[17] no doubt by tapping henequen revenue. This initiative never gained traction, leaving Mérida's poor with limited access to health care. Alvarado's collaboration with the *Junta* in support of auxiliary health units to combat smallpox stands out as one of his few effective health initiatives.

Socialist Governor Carrillo Puerto (1922–24) sought to carry revolutionary reforms much further. Carrillo Puerto had served briefly with Zapata during the Revolution and had a long history of oppositional politics—and imprisonment. He became president of the *Partido Socialista de Yucatán* when Alvarado was forced to leave the state, using the expanded party to challenge the political power of the henequen elite. The *casta divina* responded by the creation of *Asociación de Hacendados Henequeneros* (Henequen Hacendados Association), which cast its support to the Liberal Party. After a brief exile to New Orleans, Carrillo Puerto sought the governorship supported by the renamed *Partido Socialista del Sureste*, a contest he won in November 1921.

Carrillo Puerto wanted revolutionary change in Yucatán. He lacked the health care vision of Alvarado, but some rural *ligas* advocated in favor of the needs of their communities. The governor displayed considerable political skills in seeking to reform the political culture of the state however. He extended the influence of the *ligas*, supported the feminist agenda of his sister, founded new schools, and expropriated 438,000 hectares of henequen land for more than 23,000 farmers in "henequen cooperatives." The 1923 coup attempt by Adolfo de la Huerta against President Obregón reverberated through Yucatec politics, leading to Carrillo Puerto's arrest and assassination on January 3, 1924.[18] With Carrillo Puerto's death, the *Partido Socialista del Sureste* was cleansed of its most threatening social objectives. Lands were returned to henequen *hacendados* and political "normalcy" was restored to Yucatán, even as revolutionary policies were being elaborated in Mexico City.

The revolutionary Constitution of 1917 initiated the slow transformation of the Mexican state. Public health was declared to be a right of citizens, but it was quite unclear how that right was to be guaranteed. Unlike the *Consejo Superior de Salubridad*, the newly created *Departamento de Salubridad Pública* (DSP) was conceived of as a truly federal body with authority over the entire nation. DSP leader José María Rodríguez (1917–20) faced the daunting challenge of organizing the body and articulating a revolutionary vision of public health.

The establishment of Special Commission for the Eradication of Yellow Fever (1921–24) involved an unparalleled cooperation between state, federal, and international agencies.[19] At the national level, the Mexican government and the Rockefeller Foundation shared funding responsibilities for the Special Commission. Locally, Yucatec agents worked directly with Rockefeller manager Michael E. Connor; the state provided half of local operational funding, just as it had in the Liceaga campaign almost twenty years earlier. The Special Commission began operations in February 1921 with the arrival of Connor. Rojas Aguilar and a team of Yucatec physicians and inspectors conducted local operations.[20] The team employed the "intensive" anti-larval method favored by Rockefeller, a pattern of operations that would persist for years.[21] (Discussed in chapter 4) Somewhat predictably, financing provided to be one of the sources of tension.

Rojas Aguilar was central to the dispute. In 1922, federal authorities charged him with the misuse of yellow fever funds. DSP officials alleged that not only did he keep poor track of his expenditures, but that he used federal funds intended to pay for a nurse to support his personal chauffeur. Local officials disputed the allegations. M. Arechavela reminded federal officials that the state was supposed to pay half of the Sanitary Delegate's salary, and the Anti-Yellow Fever Commission the other half. By custom, the Director could use state funds for personal purposes, just as Connor had been doing. DSP officer Angel Brioso Vasconceles informed Rockefeller official Wycliffe Rose of the charges, noting that Rojas had allegedly offered to give Connor the 3,000 pesos that were missing. Connor declined, as he was unwilling to become involved in what he viewed as a local matter.[22] Several months of acrimonious investigations led Mexico City to withdraw their charges. Rojas Aguilar was replaced by Ramón Sabás Flores, but no charges were filed.[23]

The 1926 appointment of Dr. Bernardo Gastélum as chief of the DSP amplified the assertion of revolutionary authority over the states. Under Gastélum's leadership, the DSP instituted new regulations on milk and food hygiene, rebuilt the Federal Institute of Hygiene, initiated several new public health campaigns, and issued a new sanitary code. The 1926 Sanitary Code clearly subordinated state and local officials to federal authorities. It envisioned three patterns of public health administration: purely federal projects; joint federal and state efforts; and operations involving federal, state, and local actors. Thirty-two enhanced sanitary delegations were dispatched to state capitals to enforce the new guidelines.[24]

Physicians from many areas of the nation protested the new federal dictate.[25] The *Sociedad Médica Yucateca* spearheaded the defense of Yucatec authority, urging that all physicians join the body to "unite us in thought and action.[26] Local physicians petitioned Governor Torre Diaz to block the new regulations. In particular, the 1927 petition protested demands from the federal sanitary delegate that all local doctors register with the DSP and that they report all cases of communicable diseases. According to the DSP, this was in keeping with article 158 of the Federal Sanitary Code. Local doctors argued in rebuttal that the proposal was unconstitutional insofar as Article 4 of the Constitution of 1917 gave states the rights to authorize professions.[27] If the Sanitary Delegates wanted the information, they could request it from state authorities who already collected it. Moreover, the proposed registration would give rise to *curanderismo* because it would damage the faith of the patient in titled doctors, and would force up prices. Patients would abandon titled doctors and seek out *curanderos*, who had access to the same medicine but did not have to report to federal authorities.[28] Representatives of the *Junta Superior* journeyed to Mexico City to visit the Department of Public Health in an attempt to defuse tensions between two agencies.[29] Gastélum's vision of expanded federal activities fell short of his objectives, but indicated the vision of future federal operations.

The function and size of the federal delegation in Mérida nevertheless grew. In 1929, six people constituted the federal sanitary delegation: Nicolás Castellanos A. headed the body; Dr. Manuel Vallado served as the Bacteriological Assistant; Humberto Farrera as the Pharmaceutical Inspector; Professor Alvar A. González as scribe; María Medina as nurse; and Francisco Lara as helper. These delegates often acted in communities nominally under Mérida's jurisdiction. In March 1929, for example, a federal delegate in Campeche issued a complaint about pharmacists in the Yucatec towns of Tenado, Pomuch, and Hecelchacán. Castellanos was asked to inspect the facilities in these towns and report back to the *Jefe de Delegaciones Foráneas* (Chief of Exterior Delegations).[30] Similarly, federal delegates involved in the anti-malaria and yellow fever campaigns conducted multiple inspections, often fining persons for open wells, such as the 25-peso fee imposed on Gonzalo Medina in 1929.[31]

Sanitary delegates engaged in numerous outreach activities. In 1927, for example, Dr. Carlos Hoffman addressed the *Sociedad Médica Yucateca* about the anti-malaria campaign in Progreso.[32] Castellanos lectured at the "Melchor Ocampo" school on the "Infant Protection" campaign, on general hygiene, and the need for purified water.[33] He delivered similar talks at public schools in Kanasín and Muxupip.[34] The 1929 presidential campaign supported a *Servicio de Higiene Infantil* (Infant Hygiene Service) to help mothers. It focused upon preventative care, and a system of visiting nurses to teach hygiene and to monitor mothers. No *Centros de Higiene Infantil* were founded in Yucatán, but there was a subcommittee established in Progreso.[35]

Gastélum avidly supported the development of local health clinics linked with the federal government. Supported by President Plutarco Elías Calles (1924–1928), in early February 1927 Gastélum urged that state governors establish municipal health units. Ideally, these facilities would include a doctor, nurse, and sanitary inspector and would be established in each municipality in the country. The units would enforce the 1926 health code and follow many of the practices developed jointly by the DSP and the IHB of the Rockefeller Foundation.

Mexican and IHB officials had worked closely in the design of a program to improve rural health care. Dr. Miguel Bustamante, who served as a Rockefeller Fellow in 1926–28 at the Johns Hopkins University, desired a centralized network of health facilities that would attack underlying causes of high mortality rates. Bustamante expressed attentiveness to social and economic conditions that affected health. IHB officials, by contrast, favored a limited number of operations in rural communities focused upon a limited range of diseases.[36]

The DSP established the first *Unidad Sanitaria Cooperativa de Veracruz* (Cooperative Sanitary Unit of Veracruz) in May 1929 as a model for local health units. Each Sanitary Unit was served by a full-time staff of four doctors, a vet, and a sanitary engineer. They focused attention upon the control of communicable diseases; regulatory reform; child hygiene; and the improvement of water and sewage systems. While quite effective in lowering mortality rates, the unit was quite expensive. Nor did the units have the local, highly social mission envisioned by Bustamante. Still, similar units were established in Durango and Mazatlán, and in 1933 statewide units were established in Guanajuato and Querétaro. Although federal officials lent technical support to the local units, funding was the responsibility of local officials. The programs were flawed by funding shortages, a technical rather than social function—and perhaps—because local officials feared that the federal presence would damage the profitability of local physicians. The voluntary nature of this program spelled its doom.[37]

At least part of the failure stemmed from the 1926 code itself. The code envisioned a public health network that would create duplicate services by federal and state officials. It was not always clear which level of government would be responsible for certain health threats. Funding remained problematic. Federal efforts would have to be rethought, with federal funding and a clearer relationship between state and local officials.[38]

Federal sanitary efforts in Yucatán expanded in the early 1930s. Yucatec physician Mario Villamil Mendoza assumed control of Yucatán Federal Sanitary Delegation in 1931. Over the next three years, Villamil Mendoza developed three programs in Mérida, four centers of Rural Hygiene, and conducted various public health campaigns.[39] Each rural clinic housed a physician, nurse, sanitary agent, and assistant, who were responsible for basic medical services, including medical education. They also worked on various public health campaigns.[40]

The increased federal health bureaucracy sustained Yucatec resentment toward central authority. In 1933, the Federal Sanitary Delegation repeated their earlier request that all diseases be reported to their office. Yucatec physicians again expressed their willingness to share information on infectious diseases, though not the day-to-day illnesses that they treated. Again, the federal expectation was thought to imperil their job security, as *curanderos* were free from the expectation and could increase their workload.[41] "Our system produces a paradoxical effect, in that it rewards those who are not covered by the law, and hurts those who adhere to a law whose precepts were the acquisition of medical knowledge and the maintenance of their professional titles."[42] Such federal "intrusions" upon Yucatec public health authority paled in comparison with the revolutionary threats associated with the regime of Lázaro Cárdenas.

PUBLIC HEALTH AND THE REVOLUTIONARY STATE

Modernization of rural dwellers through health care and education drove many revolutionary aspirations. The efforts in the 1920s had little effect upon Yucatán, but a federal structure was being constructed that would sustain a nationwide health system by the 1940s. These would help to shape the most ambitious revolutionary projects, the construction of a rural health care network in conjunction with the creation of thousands of *ejidos* under the Cárdenas regime. These measures would place biomedicine at the heart of the Mexican state.

The Vera cruz rural "sanitary units" were the foundation for the *Servicio de Higiene Rural* (Rural Hygiene Service) created in 1931. Headed by Bustamante (1931–33), it drew upon both Mexican and Rockefeller funds, though never enough of the latter to satisfy Bustamante's objectives.[43] The decree to create *unidades sanitarios cooperativos* (cooperative sanitary units) envisioned agreements between state and federal officials to manage the sanitary units. Duplication of services was a critical concern, as were funding issues, which also required the assistance of municipalities.[44]

Coordination of public health efforts proved to be a particular challenge. An August 1934 *Ley de Coordinación de los Servicios Sanitarios Federales y Locales* (Law for the Coordination of Federal and Local Sanitary Services) sought to oversee and regulate these efforts.[45] By 1935, cooperation agreements had been reached with 14 states, often in support of rural cooperatives. Though unsuccessful in reaching an agreement with the Yucatec government, the Federal Sanitary Delegation in Mérida expanded its operations under the Cárdenas administration. As one of only two states not to have an agreement, Yucatán was the only state that did not make a financial payment to Coordinated Services. The federal government supplied all of its funding, totaling 201,665.7 pesos in 1940.[46] The delegation had two primary responsibilities:

to oversee public health campaigns and to manage rural health clinics in the corn zone.[47]

The vast land reform program of the Cárdenas presidency included a commitment to revolutionary public health. Upon assuming the presidency, Cárdenas issued an ambitious six-year plan intended to fulfill revolutionary promises to the rural sector. His general public health goals included: the coordination of federal, state, and local services; the development of rural health systems, and an expanded role of Federal Sanitary Delegations. The president was especially concerned that rural dwellers have health centers, access to clean water, sewage facilities, and training to reduce infant mortality.[48] In the president's opinion, the transformation of the countryside, including rural health programs, were crucial to the modernization of the country.

The creation of *ejido* health programs was thus central to Cárdenas' revolutionary agenda. *Ejidal* health units developed as a result of initiatives by physicians at the *Universidad Michoacana de San Nicolás de Hidalgo*. The *nicolaítas* had worked closely with Cárdenas during his gubernatorial term in linking health and social services. Dr. Jesús Díaz Barriga, secretary general of the DSP, collaborated with Enrique Arrequín Vélez, rector of the university, in establishing the first unit in the *ejido* of Zacapú in 1932. These medical units offered curative and preventative services. The Zacapú experiment, along with a parallel effort at the *ejido* of Ciudad Anáhuac, Nuevo León, established the principle that *ejido* members would pay part of the health services, either in cash or in kind. Only the poorest *ejidos* would be fully supported by the federal government. A major goal of the scientifically minded *nicolaítas* was to develop a "modern" attitude among peasants so that they might turn away from the *curanderos* who dominated the countryside and to develop a sense of responsibility for their own welfare.[49]

The First Rural Hygiene Congress led to the national extension of the *nicolaíta* initiative. Held in Morelia, Michoacán, in 1935, Barriga, Arrequín, and DSP chief Dr. José Siurob hosted the meeting. Cárdenas followed its recommendations in founding the office of "Collective Medical-Sanitary Ejidal Services" (*Servicios Médicos-Sanitarios Ejidales Colectivos)* as part of the Office of Coordinated Health Services in the States. (The name was changed to *Servicios de Higiene Rural y Medicina Social* in 1939.[50]) Secretary of Health and Assistance José Durán Córdoba identified two stages in the development of *Servicios Médicos Cooperativos Ejidales*. The experimental stage lasted for four years, from 1934 until 1938. Beginning in 1939, the consolidation stage began with three key features: (1) a focus upon zones of rural operation; (2) attentiveness to the demographic and social characteristics of different zones; and (3) a shared financial operation between the federal government and the *ejidatarios* served by the health services.[51]

Financing *ejidal* health programs limited their scope. In addition to requiring *ejido* residents to pay most of their health fees, the government determined to develop programs only in "economically active agricultural" zones. The Comarca Lagunera medical unit served as the model for the institutionalization of the rural medical cooperatives. Federal technological and administrative officials sought to enhance modern agricultural practices, especially through the *ejidal* credit bank. DSP officers believed initially that at least half of the funding should come from the *ejido* residents, a figure that they shortly increased to 70 percent.[52]

The program grew rapidly. From 36 units in 1936, it reached 104 units in 1938, and 120 units serving some 300,000 people by 1941. Officials of the service were pleased at its success, but overwhelmed by the demand by *ejido* residents for their services. Not all *ejidos* had access to the same set of services, and not all sought a revolutionary mission. Improved health access, however, was a common outcome of the campaign to transform the rural sector.[53]

The revolutionary objective of bringing modern health care to rural communities in Yucatán involved two distinct constituencies: *ejidos* in the "corn zone" in the south and east of the state; and residents of the henequen plantations in the northwest of the state. The DSP *Servicios Médicos Cooperativos Ejidales* had nominal control of both regions, though federal agents operated primarily in the corn zone under the Rural Hygiene Centers. These programs should have operated in the henequen zone as well, but, as will be seen, Yucatec elite hindered that possibility. The state government refused to sign an accord with the *Dirección General de Salubridad Federal y Servicios Sanitarios Coordinados*, fearful of federal intrusion upon Yucatec health "autonomy." Of the multiple agencies under this branch, only the Federal Sanitary Delegation had a relatively free hand, notably in various health campaigns.[54]

THE *HENEQUENEROS DE YUCATÁN*

The nationalization of henequen haciendas constituted a pressing priority for Cárdenas. The image of "enslaved" henequen laborers had tainted Yucatán's image for years; the *casta divina* had frustrated reform-minded revolutionary officials for almost as long. Cárdenas visited the state during his presidential campaign, stressing to labor groups that the transformation of the henequen zone was critical to Mexico's revolutionary progress. Cárdenas announced the expropriation of 360,436 hectares of hacienda land in August 1937, some ninety percent of the land planted in henequen in the state. Almost 23,000 laborers were the direct beneficiaries of the land reform, most of who were grouped into some 380 *ejidos*. Significantly, Cárdenas modified the original agrarian code to include not only residence *ejido* workers on the old henequen estates but salaried laborers as well.[55]

The expropriation of henequen estates appeared to have been a mortal blow to the *casta divina*. Neither the governments of Alvarado nor Carrillo Puerto had been able to seize the land of the plantation owners. The Cárdenas reform not only took land, but also offered development funds to the *ejidos* through the *Banco Nacional de Crédito Ejidal*.[56] However, the president was short of money. The land reform programs in Nuevo León and the indemnification of foreign companies for the recent oil nationalization left the treasury in distress. Cárdenas was ill-equipped to begin an aggressive public health program in Yucatán.[57]

Governor Humberto Canto Echeverría (1938–1942) promptly came to the aid of both the cash-strapped president and the displaced elite. After Cárdenas's declaration of the nationalization of the henequen estates, Canto Echeverría sought a meeting with the president. After weeks of delay, the governor and president met at Los Pinos, the presidential palace, on February 19, 1938. Two weeks later, Canto Echeverría decreed the creation of a civil organization, the *Henequeneros de Yucatán* (HOY). The organization would serve as the self-funding collective representing both private owners and *ejidos* in what was referred to as "The Great Ejido" (*El Gran Ejido*) that would coordinate the production and sale of all henequen throughout the state. The agreement stipulated that delivery of "medical service" by the HOY would include maternity and infant programs, along with programs against epidemic and endemic diseases.[58]

Though articulated in revolutionary language, the move was decidedly counter-revolutionary. The *Henequeneros* involved three sets of actors: the industrial sector (ex-hacendados); the agrarian sector (the *ejiditarios* and small holders); and the bureaucratic sector. The *Henequeneros* took control of the Ejidal Bank. Within a short period, ex-hacendados within the *Henequeneros de Yucatán* had regained control of the fiber plants, most distribution networks, and the credit bank. Profits from the industry flowed in profoundly disproportionate shares to the industrial sector of former hacendados.[59]

Governor Canto Echeverría's vision for the HOY focused primarily upon the economic and technical dimensions of the henequen industry. The agreement with the president included stipulations for health care, so that the governor soon announced the formation of a social assistance program (ASHOY) to overcome the "limitations" of the "Maya peasant." The governor said that the "ethnic character" of the Maya, their "biological defects," and their "abnormal diet" lay at the root of the social question. The ASHOY could address these racial features through programs of education, maternal care, and medical facilities. In particular, Canto envisioned a corps of medical students who would study the *ejido* residents and propose specific programs. A *Quinta de Salud de Ejidatario* (Facility for Ejidatario Health) that could serve up to 600 people would support their recommendations.[60]

On April 10, 1938, the governor reconstituted the *Departamento de Sanidad y Beneficencia*. This new body continued many of the functions of the *Junta Superior*, albeit in slightly reorganized services. Most significantly, it spoke of *Servicios sanitarios coordinados local y federal* (SSC) to coordinate federal and state health policies through ASHOY. The head of the SSC became part of the *Delegación Sanitaria Federal* in the effort to coordinate actions between the two governments.[61] Though not formalized into an agreement, it did represent linkages between the two governments, as well as adherence to revolutionary health care objectives.[62]

The apparently revolutionary social consciousness of the Department stands in stark contrast to its earlier mission. Director Carlos Mendoza Bas informed Canto Echeverría that the Department wished to "intensify" its "social labor" by bringing the benefits of "sanitary precepts" to the towns of the interior and especially to the "Mayan Indians." Mendoza intended to reorganize the Auxiliary Health Boards to make them more responsive to the mission of the Department and create new bodies in communities that lacked them; to use the medical facilities of the ASHOY as members of the expanded Auxiliary Health Boards; and to remind municipal officers that it is "their obligation to lend moral and material support to the Auxiliary Health Boards."[63]

The "Social Assistance" branch of the HOY was responsible for the delivery of health care to the *ejidos* and went far beyond the governor's vision. Mérida housed a hospital and outpatient center; the External Ejido Medical Service (*Servicio Médico Ejidal Foraneo*) operated in the henequen zone.[64] The henequen zone itself was divided into eight different sectors, each of which had a Regional Center (Category A), various Auxiliary Centers (Category B), and Rural Centers (Category C). The first of these zones to be developed, Medical Unit 1 in Acanceh, typified the range of facilities. Minor surgeries were performed at a 12 bed clinic; three nearby *ejidos* housed "B" level Sanitary Assistance Units; while "C" health stations were located in thirteen *ejidos*. Two ambulances were stationed in Acanceh to serve the various centers.[65] The "A" facilities were located in Hunucmá, Tixkokob, Motul, Cansahcab, Izamel, Acanceh, Molas, and Maxcanú. Titled physicians from nearby Auxiliary Health Boards, or physicians from Mérida staffed these units.[66] The "B" *Unidades Médicas Ambulantes* were the most important appendages of the ASHOY in the zone. Two doctors, one assistant, and two dispensary staff were part of each team that would regularly visit the *ejidos*. Each facility housed an ambulance that made regularly scheduled and emergency visits. The Category C dispensaries in the zone tended to be staffed by aids and nurses, not titled physicians.[67] By the early 1950s, 68 "A" and "B" medical dispensaries operated in the zone, plus 42 "C" infirmaries. Some 62 titled physicians; 14 medical students; 17 orthodontists; 12 surgeons; 64 dispensary staff; 32 first-level nurses; 42 second-level nurses; and a range of assistants constituted the medical staff.[68]

Facilities in Mérida served as the node of ASHOY activities. Initially, zone residents used the Hospital O'Horan. An outpatient clinic opened in Mérida in 1938 on Calle 58–519. The *Sanitario para Ejiditarios Henequeneros* (Sanitarium for Henequen Ejidatarios) opened on May 1, 1940, with forty beds for men and women. In 1941, the numbers of beds were doubled, and services were reorganized. Over the next four years, these facilities treated some 35,000 *ejiditarios* and 140,000 family members. Physicians estimated that these services reduced deaths in the henequen zone by twenty percent.[69] ASHOY officials expressed pride in the fact that a large percentage of the people who sought care at local and regional hospitals were pregnant women. Considerable efforts were undertaken to convince women through public education to use ASHOY facilities. "You have to think of the mentality of these people, who have been untouched by progress until the last few years."[70]

The *Hospital para Ejiditarios "20 de Noviembre"* was opened in 1946. From the start, doctors at the institution received people from the *ejidos* and conducted visits to the henequen zone, a fact that was reflected in the new structure. External Medicine, which received between 77,000 and 129,000 visits per year during the 1940s, became a stand-alone agency. Joining it were Services for Surgery, Otolaryngology, Ophthalmology, and Urology, and Women's Surgery and Gynecology. In the first five years of the hospital, 2,754 people were treated as inpatients.[71]

By the 1950s, the social assistance program of the *Henequeneros de Yucatán* was firmly implanted within the health care system of Yucatán. It served as the conduit for medical and pharmaceutical assistance to *ejiditarios* and their families. Eduardo L. Menéndez notes the speed in bringing medical services to the henequen zone. According to the census of 1940, of the 457 *ejidos* in region; 46 enjoyed permanent medical services; 163 had periodic service, 86 of the latter had hospital and pharmacy service.[72]

Access to ASHOY facilities expanded considerably. Initially, only *ejido* members and their families, along with the wage-laboring *parcelados* of the zone, could use the ASHOY. This access was soon expanded to employees of HOY and (in 1945) to the Agrarian Communities League (*Liga de Comunidades Agrarias*) and the *Sindicatos de Campesinos de Yucatán* (Yucatec Campensinos Syndicate). Finally, in 1952, employees of the Agrarian Department and the *Comisión de Agraria Mixta* (Mixed Agrarian Commission) gained access. This meant that some 46,000 employees and their families (two-thirds of them *ejiditarios*)—an estimated 233,000 people—had access to the ASHOY public health system. Yucatán's population in 1950 was estimated at about 519,000.[73]

Favoritism and political corruption permeated the *Henequeneros de Yucatán*, including its social assistance network of rural clinics. Scores of positions in Mérida and in the interior reduced the glut of physicians that had developed in the early 1930s. Opportunities in municipal towns no doubt alleviated the need to seek employment in Mérida, and perhaps reversed that flow. Former *hacendados* enriched themselves by their relationships to the organization, and some profited immensely. José Patrón Cervera, an intermediary between the *Henequeneros* and international purchasing houses, made millions from the sale of fiber. Rafael Salazar Trejo, an early director of the HOY, earned the nickname of the "good thief."[74] Cronyism certainly extended to the social assistance program of the HOY, especially given the large number of positions that suddenly became available during a period of economic decline. The case of Dr. Mario Erosa Cámara perhaps reveals the tip of an iceberg of corruption.

Political machinations frustrated Erosa Cámara, leading him to pen the *Epistolario de un médico*, a rare insight into the relationship between political corruption and the medical community. In 1984, Erosa Cámara published a collection of his letters written to colleagues over the years. Each letter represents a stage of his life, such as a missive to a friend with whom he attended medical school, or the transfer of the *20 de Noviembre* Hospital to the federal government in 1972.[75]

Family connections shaped Erosa Cámara's professional career. The family resided in the village of Cansahcab to the north of Ixamel, where Mario was born in 1916. His father, Vicente Erosa Leal, practiced medicine in the town, no doubt associating with Antonio Aranda, the powerful local *jefe político*. Aranda dominated the local political scene and was particularly well connected to Governor Canto Echeverría.[76] Vicente was associated with the medical program of the HOY from its founding, serving as a leader of the medical section. When father Vicente died of a heart attack in 1939, his son (also named Vicente) took Mario under his wing. Vicente worked with Enrique de Zavala y Díaz to gain Mario a post as a medical assistant at the HOY. Mario writes of his daily drives from Mérida to a series of five *ejidos*. Mario held this position until he graduated from medical school in 1943, when he was named as a consulting physician at the HOY sanitarium in Mérida. Within two years he had risen to Head of the Women's Service; a position transferred to the *20 de Noviembre* Hospital when it opened in 1946.[77] Mario studied children's health in Cuba, with a focus on mental retardation.

Brother Vicente played important roles during the gubernatorial term of José González Beytia (1946–51). He served first as Mérida's municipal president (1947–40), and then as a delegate to the state legislature (1950–52).

As soon as Vicente gained the municipal presidency, he appointed Mario head of the city's medical services, a position he held until 1953.[78] Unfortunately for the two brothers, *camarilla* politics had their downsides.

Governor González Beytia acted as director of the HOY. As his term of office neared its end, he forwarded Manuel Pasos Peniche as his successor, a logical choice given his experience in the organization. President Miguel Alemán Valdés (1946–1952) vehemently disliked Pasos Peniche however, favoring instead Campeche-born Tomás Marentes Miranda. Recognizing the power of the president, González Beytia resigned his post and went into self-imposed exile. The legislature appointed an interim governor, and signaled its dislike for Pasos Peniche. Vicente led the opposition, sponsoring anti-Marentes rallies and demonstrations. In the end, these efforts were futile, as the power of the presidential *destape* earned Marentes Miranda a six-year term as governor. These political machinations cost Vicente his job, and Mario suffered as well. After a doctor complained to the governor about him holding two jobs, Mario was dismissed from his position with municipal health services.[79]

Mario initially weathered the 1955 federalization of the ASHOY, becoming its vice-director. He attended SSA courses in Mexico City for hospital administrators, but was fired from his administrative position in 1957 in a cleansing of the "aristocrats" from the facility. Mario continued as a physician however, working with women's services until the hospital closed in 1972.[80]

Corporate paternalism permeated the health care system. Within months of the establishment of the HOY, the *Liga de Comunidades Agrarias y Sindicatos* was formed as an ally of the *Confederación Nacional de Campesinos* (National Confederation of Peasants, CNC) in the henequen zone.[81] Local residents used these linkages to appeal for additional medical services, or to complain about existing services. These petitions reflected Cárdenas's populist discourse, appealing to "revolutionary spirit" of health officials.[82] Though state health officials ran the ASHOY, corporate paternalism enabled *ejido* residents and workers to bypass Yucatán's political structures by appealing to the revolutionary regime. This facilitated new patterns of political discourse that became critical components of the emerging revolutionary state.

Ejidal commissions, Transportation Syndicates, and *Ligas de Resistencia* sought the direct influence of the president to enhance local health services. Santiago Méndez Concha, representing the Ejidal Commission of Muxip, solicited a permanent physician for his *ejido* in 1939 because they felt that HOY services were inadequate.[83] Officials of the local chapter of the National Syndicate of Public Health Workers complained that the Federal Sanitary Delegation had blocked their request to retain the nursing services of María Lucia Montes de Oca and Aurora Morales de Amaro. When the Syndicate threatened to strike because of the issue, the Sanitary Delegation in turn threatened to dissolve the local chapter.[84]

Cárdenas responded to these appeals. In November 1939, the president complained about conditions in Yucatán to José Siurob, head of the DSP. The president's recent tour of the state had revealed to him the glaring lack of services; some facilities lacked supplies, and others had no access to health care. The lack of public health services was particularly striking in indigenous communities. He ordered the DSP to develop programs of Maternity Care and Nutrition, asking that at least ten centers be including in the next budget. Sanitary officials were to work with the Department of Indian Affairs to determine appropriate communities. The federal delegation was chastised for its failure to coordinate with local officials; delegates should reach out to the state government to avoid the duplication of services.[85]

The presidential edict yielded results. Siurob informed Cárdenas that he was writing ten centers into the budget, plans that would account for about 40 percent of the proposed increase.[86] By August of 1940, at least six "Rural Hygiene Services" were to report to three regional headquarters.[87]

Yucatec syndicates and other corporate groups feared these services would end with the Cárdenas presidency. At least four groups wrote the president before he was to leave office in protest of a rumored reduction in the forthcoming health care budget. The National Syndicate of Public Health Workers (*Sindicato Nacional de Trabajadores de Salubridad Pública*) appeared to be spearheading the effort, as their telegrams from at least five towns contained the same wording.[88] Ávila Camacho was flooded with similar requests upon taking office.[89]

Even as some constituents feared for the loss of ASHOY services, state and federal cooperation slowly expanded health care in other areas. The Law of May 6, 1939, created the state *Departamento de Asistencia Social*. This section controlled the Hospital O'Horán and the Asilo Ayala, as well as the *Hospital de Niños*, then under construction with mixed state and federal funding.[90] An Infancy Protection Department (*Departamento de Protección a la Infancia*) opened in 1943, with clinics aimed at offering services to pregnant women, their newborns, and children. The Department also carried out maternal educational activities.[91]

The federal sanitary delegation benefited from the institutionalization of revolutionary health. By 1940, the delegation oversaw an epidemiological lab, an anti-TB section with three doctors; an anti-venereal section (doctor and nurse); various sanitary programs supported by twenty nurses; and anti-malaria section with 54 employees. In addition to the anti-malarial and anti-tuberculosis campaigns, the delegation managed a Center of Infant Hygiene.[92]

The federal government also maintained sanitary delegations in Celestún and Progreso as part of its *Servicio de Puertos y Fronteras*. The office in

Celestún, the smaller, older port, maintained only a sanitary delegation. In Progreso, however, the nine-person sanitary delegation oversaw campaigns against yellow fever and tropical disease, the bubonic plague, and venereal diseases.[93] The federal *Servicios Antilarvarios* operated in Progreso and Mérida; though a shortage of federal funds hindered the purchase of oil to spread on infested ponds.[94]

PUBLIC HEALTH IN THE CORN ZONE

Public health programs on *ejidos* in the corn zone developed in parallel to those of the ASHOY, though under federal auspices and with much lower funding levels. As a result, public health facilities affected fewer residents and a smaller number of communities. The federal *Servicios de Higiene Rural y Medicina Social* adhered to the "type A, B, C" model seen in the henequen zone. Centers of Rural Hygiene sought six broad objectives: public education; statistical management; sanitary engineering (with a focus on potable water); food hygiene (insured through inspections); communicable diseases; and pre-school and public school hygiene.[95] By 1940, "A" centers operated in Peto, Ticul, Tizimín, and Valladolid, each attended by a physician, nurse, sanitary agent, and helper. Each of the four centers served a "Sanitary District" of numerous *ejidos*.[96] Smaller "B" centers in Sotuta, Cenotillo, Halacho, Tekit, Tekax, and Telchac Puerto reported to the "A" centers. Nurses headed "C" level auxiliary units in ten other villages.[97]

Corn *ejidos* also worked through syndicates to resolve political struggles or administrative problems. In 1942, the Peto center was closed and moved to Tekax. Peto officials protested that the move denied them of crucial services and was politically motivated. The secretary general of the local chapter of the *Federación Ligas Gremiales Oberos y Campesinos* accused DSP officer Rafael Sánchez Centano of immoral conduct, in that the real motivations with the move lay with his quarrels with members of the Peto municipal government. Salvador Iturbide Alvárez, head of the DSP, repudiated the accusation, insisting that sanitary problems in the Tekax area necessitated the move.[98]

Ten years later funding shortages led to similar protests. A clinic had been established in Espita in 1947, with limited support from the DSP. In 1953, an auditor reported that the community needed to begin paying a 2,000 peso monthly fee, or face closure of the facility. The Syndicate League *Geronides Moguel* protested to President Ruiz Cortines, lamenting the potential loss of a now critical health post.[99] Much to their delight, the president shortly announced that the facility would stay open under SSA auspices, though the 150-member community would need to pay 78 pesos per year for the service.[100]

State officials eventually extended their operations into the corn zone through the auspices of the *Henequeneros de Yucatán*. Governor José González Beytia reported in 1948 that ASHOY clinics had been established in Muná, Santa Elena, Sotuta, Sucilá, Tunkas, and Pibtech. The clinics worked on two broad areas: public health, including sanitary, epidemiological, prenatal, and infant hygiene activities; and public assistance, including consultations, home visits, and deliveries. The governor made clear that the units sought to extend the influence of "scientific medicine," thereby protecting these communities from the actions of midwives, empirics, and *curanderos*."[101]

The Yucatec *Zona Ejidal Maicera* was one of twenty-four regional systems operated by the federal Rural Cooperative Medical Services (SMRC) in the early 1950s.[102] Director José Durán Córdoba proudly reported that nationwide the SMCR reached some 60,000 heads of families, with services offered to 315,624 people. It is unclear how many people were served in Yucatán, but it is noteworthy that ASHOY served almost 250,000 people at the same time.

Bienestar Rural

International agencies played a limited role in the development of Yucatec public health systems. The UN Program of Rural Wellbeing, created in 1953 during the presidency of Ruiz Cortines, is an exception. The Rural Wellbeing initiative envisioned a holistic approach to public health, cultural change, social well-being, and economic development. It articulated six broad goals: (1) Maternal and Infant protection; (2) Sanitation promotion; (3) Education and Cultural Promotion ("to persuade commoners not just to accept, but to actively promote the Office and its sanitary campaigns"); (4) Agricultural Development; (5) Recreation; and (6) General Activities. Typical of the increasingly bureaucratic state, representatives from the Secretaries of Government; Agriculture and Cattle Raising; Communications and Public Works; Economy; Public Education; Hydraulic Resources; and the IMSS served on Coordinated Commission on the Rural Wellbeing Program (*Comisión Coordinada del Programa de Bienestar Rural*).[103]

The Rural Wellbeing program grew quite rapidly. Six pilot Rural Wellbeing Centers were established in September 1953. That number increased to 65 by May of 1954;[104] Yucatán's first Rural Wellbeing center opened in September 1956. Five Yucatec programs were established in the next year, in Kantunil, X-Can, Tekantó, Buctzotz, and Oxkutzcab, all communities of fewer than 1500 people. Though subsidized by the federal government, most funds came from local communities that hosted the centers—as well as the land used for buildings and crops. As in the various National Indigenous Institute operations in indigenous areas, the Rural Wellbeing program relied upon local "promoters" to oversee activities. The selection process of the promoters is unclear, though many were women. The role of women in part reflects the importance of sewing and household-centered programs. Agricultural development focused upon the creation of pastures for grazing and truck gardening, especially in raising citrus trees. In Kantunil, the federal government provided some 800 citrus trees for the center. It failed, however, to fund construction of the center itself, leading the community to hold dances to raise funds.[105]

The success of promoters varied greatly. A 1958 report noted that Thelma Simá, the promoter of X-Kan, was quite enterprising, arranging for sewing lessons to be held in the homes of women who owned sewing machines until the center could purchase their own machines. By contrast, Efrén Gil Buenfil, Kantunil's promoter, complained that he had to do many visits to "change the popular impressions of promoters." A federal inspector suggested that the negative impressions might be due to his own disorganization and that the community would be better served by a new agent. In general, the inspector noted the need for additional federal funding, and a far greater emphasis upon health care, especially involving vaccinations and infectious diseases.[106]

Within a few years, the "penetration road"[107] of the Rural Wellbeing program extended to the birthing bed. The "Training Program of Empiric Midwives" sought to "control" rural midwives and to foment hygienic practices. In conjunction with the *Centro de Materno Infantil* (Infant and Maternal Center), the Rural Wellbeing centers taught rural midwives to sanitize houses, offer prenatal health care, nutrition and good septic practices.[108]

These programs sought to replace patterns of "traditional" child birth. In eastern Yucatán, this included a monthly stomach massage by a midwife to insure that the fetus was well positioned. When the woman went into labor, the midwife administered a hot tea made of mint, cinnamon, and other local herbs. Similar beverages followed a successful birth, to aid in the "ripening" of the milk. This information on "Maya midwifery" was shared with Katheryn Mackay by Gregoria Canul and Leandra Caamal, peasants who lived near the Chichen Itzá archeological site being developed by the Carnegie Institute.[109] Biomedical practitioners sought to reorient midwives to better serve their purposes in the name of national progress.

THE DECLINE OF THE *HENEQUENEROS DE YUCATÁN*

The post-World War II collapse of henequen prices bankrupted the *Henequeneros de Yucatán*, even as it had developed the nation's most complex public health system for *ejido* residents.[110] President Ruiz Cortines abolished the *Henequeneros* in 1955, nationalizing all aspects of its operations.

The *Banco Nacional de Crédito Ejidal* (BANEJIDAL) took over management of the distribution and sale of henequen, while the SSA assumed control of the social assistance facilities as part of the *Servicios Médicos Ejidales Cooperativos.*

Federal oversight through the SSA suggests the complexity of the state role in rural Mexico. Agents of BANEJIDAL worked closely with the transfer of authority, conducting technical analyses of the zone. They identified areas of the henequen zone where *Servicios Médicos Ejidales Cooperativos* would be active in conjunction with Peripheral Services (*Servicios Perifícios*) and *Bienestar Rural*, which had not been previously active in the zone.[111] SSA officials also began an infant dietary program and an antituberculosis campaign.[112] Satisfactory funding of the programs, however, remained a fundamental concern.

Ejido residents and agrarian organizations expressed grave concern that the transfer would cripple their health care facilities. The Yucatec League of Agrarian Communities (*Liga Comunidades Agrarias de Yucatán*), a powerful political force since 1938, feared that the economic crisis would lead to a suspension of public health services, threatening the well-being of some 47,000 *ejiditarios*. The organization alleged that the BANEJIDAL was bankrupt and that the SSA was not committed to the project.[113] BANEJIDAL was supposed to continue to fund the public health system by a 6 percent tax on henequen that needed to yield 800,000 pesos per year, not enough to pay for the system.[114] Nor would the *20 de Noviembre* Hospital be immune from funding shortages.[115] Already, financial distress was producing horrific conditions at Hospital O'Horan; patients could not afford to have operations, were being forced to buy their own drugs, and the institution faced a severe shortage of nurses.[116]

Multiple organizations lobbied for a financing formula that could sustain the public health system in the henequen zone. Yucatec agricultural officials wrote President Ruiz Cortines in 1956 that the system was on the verge of collapse. Large landowners in the henequen zone were threatening to withdraw their support from the public system in favor of private care. They advocated a new three-way financing system: a six centavo per kilogram tax on *ejidos* and small producers; increased payments from the fiber plants (controlled by the large owners); and greater SSA supports.[117] An accord was finally reached in early 1958 in which BANEJIDAL agreed to oversee a tax on henequen production that would yield 3.8 million pesos annually; SSA would be responsible for 200,000 pesos. With this funding, the *Servicios Médicos Rurales Cooperativos* would be able to continue existing medical services.[118] Within months, however, local officials warned of that the budget shortfall would reach half-million pesos, funds that would have to come from the SSA which was short of funding.[119]

Twenty years after the establishment of the HOY, President Cárdenas reflected on the shortcomings of the ASHOY. In a 1957 visit to Yucatán, Cárdenas echoed the complaints of the *ejiditarios*. Even though his administration had established the policy that *ejido* residents should pay for most of the health services on the ejidos, the president now expressed deep regrets. Over the years, residents had paid for the physicians and the social assistance program. "This situation is unjust by any degree of thought; it lowers the income of the *ejidatarios* and reduces the quality of the medical services that they can afford."[120] Unfortunately, the national reality was worse. Just over 18 million Mexicans in 1957 lived in rural environments. The federal *Servicios Médicos Rurales Cooperativos* reached 1,398,296 residents, just thirteen percent of rural Mexicans.[121] Cárdenas's revolutionary aspirations of bringing "modern" health care to rural dwellers had not come to pass, save perhaps in Yucatán, where the collapse of henequen prices now threatened its well-being.

ASSESSING REVOLUTIONARY PUBLIC HEALTH

By the late 1950s, the federal government dominated public health activities in much of Yucatán. Especially in rural areas—in both the corn and henequen zones—the federal government had supplanted the activities of the state government. The SSA managed rural systems through the *Servicios Médicos Rurales Cooperativos*, with a Regional Center in Mérida; five auxiliary centers in Valladolid, Tekax, Ticul, Tizimín, and Motul; and thirteen rural centers. Public health campaigns continued against yellow fever, malaria, maternal and infantile health, and tuberculosis.

A nationwide inspection in 1957 offers a rare overview of public health programs in Yucatán. Officials from the *Secretaria de Salubridad y Asistencia* ordered inspectors to visit every state and territory, seeking to determine the effectiveness of federal health programs throughout the country. Julio Viniegra Villalba investigated the two federal programs in Yucatán, the newly established *Bienestar Rural* and the long-active federal sanitary delegations. Viniegra Villalba reported that the delegation divided its operation into six sectors within the corn zone, managed from the central office in Mérida. Other zones were centered in Progreso, Tekax, Ticul, Valladolid, and Tizimín. Five *Bienestar Rural* centers had been in operation for fewer than six months in Kantunil, X-can, Tekantó, Buctzotz, and Oxkutzcab. Viniegra Villalba noted that while none of these programs collaborated directly with Yucatec agencies, "cordial" relations existed between state and federal officials in most areas.[122]

Despite an extensive public health infrastructure that covered much of Yucatán, the inspector issued a negative report card. The six zones managed by the federal sanitary delegation suffered from a lack of funding, poorly organized services, inadequate facilities, and weak personnel. Programs were supposed to receive at least thirty percent of the budget, but over ninety percent of the budget went to salaries. As a result, programs such as the Mother-Child Hygiene Center, dispensaries to combat tuberculosis, venereal disease, skin disease, and the visiting nurses were largely ineffective. Viniegra Villalba made few positive comments, reserving praise only for the laboratory in Mérida and the newly reorganized (1951) center in Progreso. He recommended that all centers be given vehicles so that they could expand their services, that all facilities should be upgraded and—most importantly—that they needed "EFFECTIVE, EXPANDED, AND DIRECTED COORDINATION."[123]

Malnutrition, illness, and various imbalances characterized the region. The critical imbalances centered on the henequen zone, and were visible in both demographic patterns and in terms of public health investment. Including the capital city, the henequen zone contained almost 64 percent of the population despite occupying only 22 percent of the land. The corn and cattle zones comprised 43 percent of the territory and 30 percent of the population, while the remaining seven percent of the state's residents occupied the forest and coastal areas of the remaining third of the territory. The henequen zone had long enjoyed *Banco Ejidal* funds, so that almost 95 percent of the 24 million pesos spent on health services by the SSA went to the henequen zone and Mérida. The rest of the residents had scant access to health care and limited funding.[124]

The final collapse of the henequen industry deprived the state of its economic dynamo. Still, a 1959 investigation promised that Yucatán remained a "privileged region." Maya ruins and the lure of "folklore" highlighted the tremendous tourist potential of the region. Lacking were roads, hotels, and other necessities for the tourist trade. For this potential to be realized, the CINEPY team concluded that "health and welfare" investments constituted the fundamental building blocks for the future.[125]

The CINEPY team linked health care to the future development of the state. To begin, it would be necessary to achieve demographic and health care balance in the region. About half of the families in the henequen zone needed to move into more economically viable areas. SSA funds needed to be invested more evenly throughout the state, and new funds were needed for seven new Centers for Integrated Health. Gastrointestinal diseases, the region's primary health problem, would be addressed by the investment of over 70 million pesos in wells, latrines, and water pipes. The Rural Wellbeing programs were to be expanded, once again linking agricultural, human, and health concerns—locating public health programs firmly within plans for economic development. Another 77 million pesos should be invested in rural education. Finally, the administration of health care services needed to be

Table 5.1 Yucatec public health clinic expansion, 1957–1963

	Municipalities	*No. of clinics*
1957	106	14
1958	106	38
1959	106	39
1960	106	49
1963	106	76

Source: M. E. Bustamante, "La coordinación de los servicios sanitarios federales y locales como factor de progreso higiénico en México, su evolución y desarrollo de 1934 a 1964," in *Libro conmemorativo del Primer Centenario, Academic Nacional de Medicina,* Tomo II (México DF: Academic Nacional de Medicina, 1964), 654.

reformed (the seven different agencies active in the state were judged to lack coordination) and their emphasis needed to be redirected toward sanitation and preventative medicine.[126]

A burst of construction in the early 1960s both updated and expanded the federal health network in Yucatán. President Adolfo López Mateos (1958-1964) inaugurated eight new facilities in January 1962, one-fifth of the new centers that would be opened by the end of his administration two years later. A large majority of these were in the henequen zone, though updates had been made in the corn zone and capital of Mérida as well. Included in these projects were 18 Centers for Primary Care for Mothers and Infants, and a tuberculosis wing at the *20 de Noviembre* Hospital. The bulk of the new centers adhered to a similar layout of some 400 square meters that took about three months to construct and were intended to serve smaller communities. It was estimated by locating the centers in towns of 2,000 or so people, more than twice that number of people would now have access to health care.[127]

CONCLUSION

The roles of the Yucatec and revolutionary regimes in the development of public health systems in Yucatán were complementary and contested. The governments shared a common ideology of the modernizing function of public health, so that either might articulate the progressive benefit of biomedical care. Henequen profits drove the Yucatec state to isolate rural laborers and hacendados from "outside" influences, especially revolutionaries who sought to bring these critical industries under state control (and transform rural health care in the process). Yucatec efforts to stifle revolutionary change in henequen power relations led to the development of one of Mexico's most complete rural health care systems, a process that brought the state into the day-to-day lives of rural residents. The weakness of the henequen economy, not the strength of the revolutionary state, reduced Yucatán's control over its own system of public health.

As Miguel E. Bustamante reflected in 1964 on the evolution of Mexico's public health system during his long and distinguished career, he highlighted the fundamental changes brought by the Revolution. Methodical programs of social assistance had replaced earlier notions beneficence, and an overarching and a global sense of the social function of public health had replaced limited conceptualizations of hygiene; together, they had led to a substantial reduction in rates of mortality throughout the country. Bustamante thought that the industrial sector had made much greater progress than the rural sector, but infrastructure improvements, agricultural technology, and a greater openness to biomedical practices had improved the health of Mexico's rural population.[128]

Absent from Bustamante's analysis is a sense of the transformed political culture that sustained Mexico's public health system. If a rural resident in 1910 Yucatán had sought assistance from a biomedical healer, he or she would have to seek out a political patron for referral to Hospital O'Horan in Mérida. Few biomedical physicians lived outside the capital, so that political connections were the only alternative to traditional healers. Forty years later, with the development of ASHOY and the federal rural health centers in the corn zone, biomedical health care had become ruralized and accessible to most residents. Complaints or appeals for greater services would be channeled through *ejido* organizations, often directly linked to the corporate structure of the revolutionary state. New forms of claim-making—through telegrams, petitions, or letters—linked most rural dwellers to an increasingly bureaucratized revolutionary state, often bypassing Yucatec officials. The construction of new clinics in small communities by the SSA and IMSS evidenced the increased influence of the revolutionary center, and the marginalization of the once powerful Yucatec state.

NOTES

1. Pedro Castillo Cervera (federal delegate in Progreso) to Alfonso Pruneda, Progreso, July 3, 1922, ASSHA, Sección Oficialia Major, Caja 1, exp. 12; Pruneda to Governor of State, Mexico City, July 20 1922, ibid.

2. Departamento de Salubridad Pública, *Los servicios de higiene rural y medicina social* (México DF: Artes Gráficos del Estado, S. C. I., 1941), 15.

3. Elise Rockwell, "Schools of the Revolution: Enacting and Contesting State Forms in Tlaxcala, 1910–1930," in *Everyday Forms of State Formation: Revolution and the Negotiation of Rule in Modern Mexico*, ed. by Gilbert M. Joseph and Daniel Nugent (Durham: Duke University Press, 1994), 173–74.

4. A rich literature on Mexican state formation has developed in recent years. Central to that literature are the essays in *Everyday Forms of State Formation.* Other important contributions include Nora Hamilton, *The Limits of State Autonomy: Post-Revolutionary Mexico* (Princeton: Princeton University Press, 1982). In the realm of medicine, please see Gustavo Nigenda-López, *The Medical Profession, the State and Health Policy in Mexico,* 1917–1988 (D. Phil. London School of Economics and Political Science, 1995); James Angus McLeod, *Public Health, Social Assistance, and the Consolidation of the Mexican State,* 1888–1940 (Ph. D. diss., Tulane University, 1990); and McCrea, *Diseased Relations.*

5. Birn, *Marriage of Convenience*, 44.

6. Ana María Carrillo, "Economía, política y salud pública en el México porfiriano (1876–1910)," *História, Ciência, Saúde—Manguinhos* 9 (202), 67–87.

7. Carrillo, "Los difíciles caminos," 21; Birn, *Marriage of Convenience*, 44–45; Claudia Agostoni, *Monuments of Progress: Modernization and Public Health in Mexico City,* 1876–1910 (Calgary: University of Calgary Press, University Press of Colorado, Instituto de Investigaciones Históricas, UNAM, 2003).

8. Fernando Martínez Cortés and Xóchitl Martínez Barbosa, *El Consejo Superior de Salubridad. Rector de Salud Pública en México* (México: SmithKline Beecham Mexico, 1997), 32–34.

9. Carrillo, "Economía, política y salud pública."

10. McLeod, *Public Health, Social Assistance, and the Consolidation of the Mexican State,* 1888–1940, 43–44.

11. Francisco C. Cárdenas (Jefe del Servicio especial contra la fiebre amarilla) to President of the Consejo Superior de Salubridad, Mérida, February 6, 1908; ibid, February 26, 1908, ASSHA, FSP, Sección Epidemiologia, Caja 7, exp. 7; Cárdenas to Educardo Liceaga, Mérida, December 31, 1906, ASSHA, FSP, Sección Epidemiologia, Caja 5, exp. 5; Enrique Múñoz Arístequi to Liceaga, February 4, April 17, June 12, June 19, 1907, ibid.; Liceaga to Múñoz, Mexico City, April 24, 1907, May 13, 1907, ibid.

12. Sec. of the Departamento de Salubridad Pública to Jefe de Hacienda of the state of Yucatán, Mexico City, July 26, 1922, ASSHA, FSP, Sección Epidemiología, Caja 30, exp. 10.

13. Gustavo Vega to Governor, April 16, 1914, Mérida, AGEY, JPE, Sec. Beneficencia, Series Correspondencia, Sanidad, 1914, Caja 453.

14. Birn, *Marriage of Convenience*, 45–46.

15. Allen Wells and Gilbert M. Joseph, *Summer of Discontent, Seasons of Upheaval: Elite Politics and Rural Insurgency in Yucatán,* 1876–1915 (Stanford: Stanford University Press, 1996), 277–85.

16. Michael J. Gonzáles, *The Mexican Revolution,* 1910–1940 (Albuquerque: University of New Mexico Press, 2002), 167–71.

17. Decree of August 6, 1915, Gobierno de Salvador Alvarado, Mérida, AGEY, JPE, Sec. Beneficencia, Series Correspondencia, Sanidad, 1914, Caja 478.

18. Sergio Quezada, *Breve historia de Yucatán* (México: El Colegio de México, 2001), 194–206.

19. "Report of the Director of the Comisión Especial para la Campaña Contra la Fiebre Amarilla," RAC, RG 5, Series 323, Box 33, Folder 195; Birn, *Marriage*

of Convenience, 5–57. See also Sowell, "The Eradication of Yellow Fever in Yucatán: The Rockefeller Foundation and the Question of a Revolutionary Center" (forthcoming); Armando Solarzano, "The Rockefeller Foundation in Revolutionary Mexico: Yellow Fever in Yucatán and Veracruz," in Marcos Cueto, ed. *Missionaries of Science: The Rockefeller Foundation and Latin America* (Bloomington: Indiana University Press, 1994), 52–71; McCrea, *Diseased Relations*, 171–89.

20. Connor, "Notes on Yellow Fever in Mexico," October 15, 1923, Mérida, RAC, RG 5.2 (IHB Special Reports), Box 33, Series 323, Folder 193; ASSHA, FSP, Sección Epidemiologia, Caja 17, exp. 3; Gil Rojas to Alfonso Pruneda, Mérida, April 2, 1921.

21. Diego Hernández F. to Roberto Medellín, Jefe DSP, Mérida, December 20, 1924, ASSHA, FSP, Sección Salubridad en Territorios, Puertos y Fronteras, Caja 3, Exp. 12.

22. Angel Brioso Vasconceles to Rose, August 13, 1922, Mexico City; Connor to White, September 8, 1922, Mérida; RAC, RG 5.1.2 Box 137, Folder 1823.

23. The correspondence is located in ASSHA, FSP, Sección Epidemiología, Caja 30, exp. 10.

24. Birn, *Marriage of Convenience*, 99, 103, 119.

25. Birn, *Marriage of Convenience*, 119.

26. *La Revista Médica de Yucatán*, November 1926.

27. Article 4 stipulates: "No person can be prevented from engaging in the profession, industrial or commercial pursuit, or occupation of his choice, provided it is lawful. The exercise of this liberty shall only be forbidden by judicial order when the rights of third parties are infringed, or by administrative order, issued in the manner provided by law, when the rights of society are violated. No one may be deprived of the fruits of his labor except by judicial decision.

The law in each state shall determine the professions which may be practiced only with a degree, and set forth the requirements for obtaining it and the authorities empowered to issue it." http://www.latinamericanstudies.org/mexico/1917-Constitution.htm (accessed March 11, 2011).

28. AGEY, FPE, Sec. Beneficencia, Ser. JSS, May 23, 1927; AGEY, FPE, Sec. Beneficencia, Ser. JSS, Caja 9, exp. 40, 1929.

29. *Informe rendido al gobernador constitucional de Yucatán c. Dr. Alvaro Torre Díaz, ante la XXX Legislatura del Estado el 1° de Enero de 1928* (Mérida: Talleres Tipográficos del Gobierno del Estado, 1928), 50–51.

30. Abraham Ayala González to Nicolás Castellanos A. March 20, 1929, AHSSA, Fondo Salubridad Pública, Sección Salubridad en Territorios, Puertos y Fronteras (STPF), Caja 12, Expediente 9; N. Castellanos to Departamento de Salubridad Pública, December 27, 1929, ibid. Castellanos to A. Ayala G., Mérida, December 27, 1929, ASSHA, FSP, Sec. Salubridad en Territorios, Puertos y Fronteras, Caja 12, Exp. 9.

31. Armando Escalante G. (jefe de servicio) to Jefe DSP, Mérida April 22, 1929, ASSHA, FSP, STPF, Caja 9, Exp. 22.

32. *La Revista Médica de Yucatán*, December 20, 1927.

33. Castellanos A. (Sanitary delegate) to Ayala González (Jefe, DSP), Mérida, June 17, 1929, AHSSA, FSP, Sección Presidencia, Serie Secretaria, Caja 12, exp. 3.

34. Castellanos to Ayala González, Mérida, June 28, 1929, AHSSA, FSP, Sección Presidencia, Serie Secretaria, Caja 12, exp. 3.

35. Departamento de Salubridad Pública, *Informe general*, 9, 11.

36. Birn, *Marriage of Convenience*, 123–25.

37. Birn, *Marriage of Convenience*, 119–20, 32–37.

38. Birn, *Marriage of Convenience*, 120.

39. http://www.salud.yucatan.gob.mx/coordenfermeria.htm. Accessed August 10, 2006.

40. Departamento de Salubridad Pública, Directorio General, *La Oficina Central de Higiene Rural y Servicios Coordinados en los estados* (Mexico: Talleres del Imp. del Departamento de Salubridad Pública, 1937), 64; http://www.salud.yucatan.gob.mx/coordenfermeria.htm. Accessed August 10, 2006.

41. *La Revista Médica de Yucatán*, February 1933.

42. *La Revista Médica de Yucatán*, February 1933.

43. Birn, *Marriage of Convenience*, 142–44.

44. "Reglamentos estudios y proyectos de convenios para la creación de las unidades sanitarios cooperativos," 1931, AHSSA, FSP, Sección Jurídico, Caja 28, exp. 14.

45. M. E. Bustamante, "La coordinación de los servicios sanitarios federales y locales como factor de progreso higiénico en México, su evolución y desarrollo de 1934 a 1964," in *Libro conmemorativo del Primer Centenario, Academic Nacional de Medicina*, Tomo II (México DF: Academic Nacional de Medicina, 1964), 653.

46. Dirección de Servicios Sanitarios Coordinados en los Estados y Territorios,. *Directorio General, 1940*, Archivo General de la Nación (AGN), Fondo Lázaro Cárdenas del Río (LCR), CAJA 185, 425.5/179, April 2, 1940.

47. Dirección General de Salubridad Federal y de los Servicios Sanitarios Coordinados, "Informe sintetico de las labors desarrolladas durante el presente año comprended 1° de Septiembre de 1941 al 30 de Junio de 1942," August 4, 1942, 37–38.

48. McLeod, *Public Health, Social Assistance, and the Consolidation of the Mexican State*, 158; Birn, *Marriage of Convenience*, 177–79.

49. José Durán Córdova, *Organización y funcionamiento de los Servicios Médicos Cooperativos Ejidales* (México DF, 1951) (Mimeograph prepared for a meeting of the Asociación Fronteriza México-Norteamericano de Salubridad Pública, Los Angeles, CA.), 2; Ana María Kapelusz-Poppi, "Physician Activists and the Development of Rural Health in Postrevolutionary Mexico," *Radical History Review* 80 (Spring 2001), 36, 41–43; Kapelusz-Poppi, "Rural Health and State Construction in Post-Revolutionary Mexico: The Nicolaita Project for Rural Medical Services," *The Americas* 58:2 (October 2001), 261–83; Birn, *Marriage of Convenience*, 216–20.

50. Departamento de Salubridad Pública, *Los servicios de higiene rural y medicina social* (México DF: Artes Gráficos del Estado, S. C. I., 1941), 3, 6.

51. Durán Córdova, *Los Servicios Médicos Cooperativos Ejidales*, 2, 3, 8.

52. Secretaria de Salubridad y Asistencia, Dirección General de los Servicios Médicos Rurales Cooperativos, *Organización y funcionamiento de los Servicios Médicos Rurales Cooperativos* (México DF: SSA, 1951), 8–12; Departamento de Salubridad Pública, *Memoria, correspondiente al period septiembre* 1° de 1942–Agosto 31 de 1943 (México DF: Talleres Tipográficos Modelos, S. A., 1943), 192, 242.

53. Kapelusz-Poppi, "Physician Activists," 43–44: Menéndez, *Poder, estratificación y salud*, 245; Durán Córdova, *Organización y funcionamiento de los Servicios Médicos Cooperativos Ejidales*, 2.

54. Departamento de Salubridad Pública, *Memoria, correspondiente al period septiembre 1° de 1942-Agosto 31 de 1943*, 192, 208–15.

55. Enrique Montalvo Ortega and Iván Vallado Fajardo, *Yucatán: Sociedad, economía, política, cultura* (México DF: Universidad Nacional Autónoma de México, 1997), 28–29; Hamilton, *The Limits of State Autonomy*, 134, 166, 169.

56. Montalvo Ortega, Enrique and Iván Vallado Fajardo, *Yucatán: Sociedad, economía, política, cultura* (México DF: Universidad Nacional Autónoma de México, 1997), 23–29.

57. Viviane Brachet de Márquez, *The Dynamics of Domination: State, Class, and Social Reform in Mexico,* 1910–1990 (Pittsburgh: University of Pittsburgh Press, 1994), 77; Fallaw, *Cárdenas Compromised*, 126–27.

58. *La nueva estructura económica de Yucatán. Consideraciones, documentos y hechos relacionados con la más trascendenta obra de la revolución en materia agraria. Genesis y formación de "Henequeneros de Yucatán*" (México DF: Editorial "Al Servicio del Pueblo," 1938), 27–28; Humberto Canto Echeverría to Lázaro Cárdenas, Mérida, February 11, March 3, 1938, AGN, LCR, Caja 17, 111/856.

59. Montalvo Ortega and Vallado Fajardo, *Yucatán: Sociedad, economía, política, cultura*, 29–31. Nora Hamilton suggests that Cárdenas cooperated with the counter-revolutionary move because his government could not meet the costs associated managing the henequen industry. *Limits of State Autonomy*, 175.

60. *La nueva estructura económica de Yucatán*, 19.

61. Carlos Mendoza Bas to the Judge of the 2nd State District, May 4, 1939, AGEY, FPE, Fondo JSS, Serie Copiador de Oficios, Vol. 188, No. 154.

62. *Informe del Sr. Ingeniero Humberto Canto E., Gobernador Constitucional de Yucatán ante la XXIV legislatura del estado 1939* (Mérida: Imprenta del Estado, 1940), 20, 81.

63. Carlos Mendoza Bas to the Governor, May 25, 1939, AGEY, FPE, Sección JSS, Vol. 188, No. 362.

64. *Informe del Ciudadano Profesor José Gutiérrez Beytia, Gobernador Constitucional del Estado, año de 1948* (Mérida: Gobierno del Estado de Yucatán, 1949), 109–12.

65. *Memoria de la Secretaría de Salubridad y Asistencia Pública. Sexenio* 1952–1958 (Mexico DF: Impreso for ACMEX, S. A., 1958), 520, 532; Henequeneros de Yucatán, *Informe del Consejo Directorio de Henequeneros de Yucatán correspondiente de ejercicio de 1950* (Mérida: Editorial "Zamna," 1950), 44.

66. Samuel Aguilar Sarmiento, *La asistencia social en el ejido henequenero de Yucatán* (Mérida: NP, 1953), 10.

67. *Memoria,* 1946–1951, *Departamento de Asistencia Social de Henequeneros de Yucatán* (Mérida: Henequeneros de Yucatán, 1952), 115–16.

68. Samuel Aguilar Sarmiento, *La asistencia social en el ejido henequenero de Yucatán* (Mérida: NP, 1953), 10; *Informe de Señor Ernesto Novelo Torres Gobernador constitucional de Yucatán ante la XXXVI Legislatura del Estado, 1944* (Mérida: Imprenta del Estado, 1945), 46–48.

69. *Clinica Médico-quirúrgica* 1:6 (1944), 152.

70. *Memoria,* 1946–1951, 52–53.

71. Henequeneros de Yucatán, *Informe del Consejo Directorio de Henequeneros de Yucatán correspondiente de ejercicio de 1950* (Mérida: Editorial "Zamna," 1950), 44.

72. Menénez, *Poder estratificación y salud,* 245.

73. Aguilar Sarmiento, *La asistencia social,* 1–3.

74. Sergio Quezada, *Breve historia de Yucatán* (México: El Colegio de México, 2002), 229–31; Margaret Goodman, "Does Political Corruption Really Help Economic Development: Yucatán, Mexico," *Polity* 7:2 (Winter 1974), 143–64.

75. Mario Erosa Cámara, *Epistolario de un médico* (Mérida: Maldonado Editores, 1984).

76. Fallaw, *Cárdenas Compromised,* 52, 140–41.

77. Erosa Cámara, *Epistolario de un médico,* 38–44, 56.

78. Erosa Cámara, *Epistolario de un médico,* 56.

79. Erosa Cámara, *Epistolario de un médico,* 49–56.

80. Erosa Cámara, *Epistolario de un médico,* 59–69, 76.

81. Othon Baños Ramírez, "Contradicciones del ejido que se institucionalizó: (La Laguna y zona henequenero de Yucatán," in *Campesinos y sociedad: Ayer y hoy,* compiled by Othon Baños Ramírez (Mérida: Ediciones de Universidad Autónoma de Yucatán, 1992) 142.

82. Porfirio Mis, Ines Tun, Pablo Canul, Basilio Canul to Cárdenas, Quinta Iturralde, August 5, 1937, AGN, LCR, Caja 158, 151.3/452.

83. Santiago Méndez Concha to Cárdenas, November 22, 1939, AGN, LCR, Caja 185, 425.5/39.

84. Sindicato Nacional de Trabajadores de Salubridad Pública (Sección Estatal 13) to Lázaro Cárdenas, Mérida, August 20, 1938, AGN, LCR, Caja 185, 425.5/39.

85. Cárdenas to José Siurob, Mérida, November 25, 1939, AGN, LCR, Caja 185, 425.5/39.

86. Siurob to Cárdenas, México DF, December 30, 1939, AGN, LCR, Caja 1064, 568.2/9.

87. Aurelio Collado to Directores de los Servicios Coordinados de Salud Pública en los Estados y Territorios, México DF, August 17, 1940, AGN, Fondo Secretaría de Salubridad y Asistencia, Sección Departamento de Salubridad Pública, Caja 10 (vieja) 939 (actual).

88. A. Pacheco L, Sección 13, Delegación 1, Sindicato Nacional de Trabajadores de Salubridad Pública to Cárdenas, Ticul, November 9, 1940, AGN, LCR, 568.2/9. Also signed by delegates from the Sindicato de Carritilleros, Ministerio Público, Comisariado Ejidal de Ticul. The telegrams came from Valladolid, Tekax, Peto, Oxkutzcab, and Toluca.

89. See Caja 382 of the AGN, Fondo Manuel Ávila Camacho (MAC), 425.5/4 and 425.5/43 for the letters and telegrams.

90. *El Hospital del Niños* (Mérida: Gobierno del Estado de Yucatán, 1940).

91. *Informe de Señor Ernesto Novelo Torres Gobernador constitucional de Yucatán ante la XXXVI Legislatura del Estado, 1944* (Mérida: Imprenta del Estado, 1945), 61.

92. José F. Diaz and Benjamín Gongora Triay, "La higiene," in *Enciclopedia Yucatenense* (México DF: Edición Oficial del Gobierno de Yucatán, 1977), vol. VI, 420; Departamento de Salubridad Pública, *Directorio General, La Oficina Central de Higiene Rural y Servicios Sanitarios Coordinados en los Estado*s (NP: 1937), 64.

93. Departamento de Salubridad Pública, *La Oficina Central de Higiene Rural y Servicios Coordinados en los estados*, 66, 69; Román Sabas Flores to Jefe DSP, Progreso, October 1, 1930, ASSHA, FSP, Seccíon Salubridad en Territorios, Puertos y Fronteras (STPF), Caja 12, Exp. 9.

94. Departamento de Salubridad Pública, *Informe general*, 48–49.

95. Dirección de Servicios Sanitarios Coordinados en los Estados y Territorios. *Directorio General, 1940*, AGN, LCR, CAJA 185, 425.5/179, April 2, 1940.

96. http://www.salud.yucatan.gob.mx/coordenfermeria.htm accessed August 10, 2006.

97. Aurelio Collado to Directores de los Servicios Coordinados de Salud Pública en los Estados y Territorios, México DF, August 17, 1940, AGN, Fondo Secretaría de Salubridad y Asistencia, Sección Departamento de Salubridad Pública, Caja 10 (vieja) 939 (actual); *Directorio General, 46.* Monitoring the activities of the Rural Centers is hampered by frequent name changes. In 1946, the DSP created the *Dirección General de Higiene Rural y Medicina Social*, which oversaw the *Oficina de Servicios Médicos Ejidales*. In 1948, it became the *Dirección Generales de Servicios Rurales Cooperativos.*

98. Maximo E. Sabido to Manuel Ávila Camacho, Peto, May 7, 1942, Salvador Iturbide Alvárez to Secretary General de Federación Ligas Gremiales Oberos y Campesinos, México DF, May 27, 1942; Luis A. Ramírez Aznar to Ávila Camacho, Peto, April 27, 1944, AGN, MAC, Caja 382, 425.5/82.

99. Manual J. Dzil and Gustavo Arco V. (pres. and sec of Liga Sindical "Geronides Moguel") to Adolfo Ruiz Cortines, Espita, August 22, 1953, AGN, Fondo Adolfo Ruiz Cortines (ARC), Caja 424 425/14.

100. Prudencio Patrón Peniche to Ruiz Cortines, Espita, November 25, 1954, AGN, ARC, Caja 424 425/14.

101. *Informe del Ciudadano Profesor José Gutiérrez Beytia, Gobernador Constitucional del Estado, año de 1948* (Mérida: Gobierno del Estado de Yucatán, 1949), 80–81.

102. José Durán Córdova, *Organización y funcionamiento de los Servicios Médicos Cooperativos Ejidales* (México DF, 1951) (Mimeograph prepared for a meeting of the Asociación Fronteriza México-Norteamericano de Salubridad Pública, Los Angeles, CA.), 2, 3, 8; Secretaria de Salubridad y Asistencia, Dirección General de los Servicios Médicos Rurales Cooperativos, *Organización y funcionamiento de los Servicios Médicos Rurales Cooperativos* (México DF: SSA, 1951), 15, 18.

103. *Memoria de la Secretaría de Salubridad y Asistencia Social pública. Sexenio* 1952–1958 (México DF: Impreso por ACMEX, S. A., 1958), 459; ["Inspection report,]" ASSHA, FSSA, Sección Subsecretaría de Salubridad y Asistencia, Caja 53, expediente 3; *Diario Oficial*, October 28, 1954.

104. José Fiqueroa Ortíz, "Informe de actividades llevadas a cabo del 1° de Septiembre de 1953 al 31 de Diciembre de 1954," ASSHA, Fondo Secretaría de Salubridad y Asistencia (FSSA), Sección Subsecretaría de Salubridad y Asistencia (SSSA), Caja 51, Expediente 2 (1955), 1–3, 6.

105. ASSHA, FSSA, SSSA, Caja 53, expediente 3.

106. ASSHA, FSSA, SSSA, Caja 53, expediente 3, 2, 3, 4.

107. The Mexican Institute for Indigenous Affairs used local "promoters" to gain acceptance in local communities, a strategy they referred to as "Penetration roads." See Robert Charles Harman, *Cambios médicos y sociales en una comunidad maya-tzeltal* (México: Instituto Nacional Indigenista y Secretaría de Educación Pública, 1974).

108. ASSHA, FSSA, SSSA, Caja 55, exp. 5.

109. George Cheever Shattuck and Joseph C. Bequaert, *The Peninsula of Yucatán, Medical, Biological, Meteorological and Sociological Studies* (Washington: Carnegie Institution of Washington, 1933), 64–67.

110. In 1958, eight of the nation's 27 category "A" regional centers were in Yucatán; seventeen of the 29 category B centers were in the henequen zone, as were 75% of the category C facilities. *Memoria de la Secretaría de Salubridad y Asistencia Pública. Sexenio*, 520.

111. Secretaría de Salubridad y Asistencia, "Informe de las actividades desarrolladas por esta dependencia durante el period comprendido del 1° de Septiembre de 1954 al 31 de Agosto de 1955," ASSHA, FSSA, SSSA, Caja 48, Expediente 3, p. 6/7.

112. Secretaria de Salubridad y Asistencia. "Cuarto Informe" [1° Septiembre 1955—August 1956] [compiled by Alberto Craviolo Meneses], FSSA, Sección Subsecretaría de Salubridad y Asistencia, Caja 48, Expediente 3, 8–9.

113. Alvaro Palma Prieto to Ruiz Cortines, Mérida, December 7, 1955, AGN, ARC, Caja 424; Arturo Luna Lugo (Sec. General of the CNC) to Ruiz Cortines, December 16, 1955, México DF, AGN, ARC, Caja 426; Baños Ramírez, *Campesinos y sociedad,* 134–35.

114. Gilberto Flores Múñoz (Secretario de Agricultura y Ganadería) to Arturo Luna Lugo, México DF, December 23, 1955, AGN, ARC, Caja 426 425.1/149.

115. Alvaro Vivas Marfil (Presidente Bloque de Constituyentes del Partido Socialista del Sureste) to Ruiz Cortines, Mérida, June 21, 1955, AGN, ARC, Caja 426 425.1/133, AGN, ARC, Caja 426 425.1/149.

116. Rafael Heredia Irigoyen to Adolfo Ruiz Cortines, Mérida, June 24, 1955, AGN, ARC, Caja 426 425.1/149.

117. Miguel Serrano Gómez and Pech Tec to Ruiz Cortines, Mérida, August 23, 1956, AGN, ARC, Caja 426, 425.1/149.

118. AGN, Fondo Secretaría de Salubridad y Asistencia, Sección Dirección General de Servicios Coordinados de Salud Pública en los Estados y Territorios, Vol. 3 (viejo) 589 (actual).

119. Serrano Gómez and Tec to Ruiz Cortines, Mérida, August 15, 1958, and Arturo Cabañas Franco (Presidente Consejo Campesino) to Ruiz Cortines, Mérida, August 15, 1958, both in AGN, ARC, Caja 424.

120. Cárdenas, "Reparto agrario viente años despues," September 10, 1957, in *Lázaro Cárdenas en Yucatán (1934–1957): Discursos.*

121. *Memoria de la Secretaría de Salubridad y Asistencia Pública. Sexenio*, 511.

122. The reports are located in the ASSHA, FSSA, SSSA, Caja 53, expediente 3.

123. Capitalization in the original. ASSHA, FSSA, SSSA, Caja 53, expediente 3.

124. Comisión Intersecretarial para el estudio de los Problemas de Yucatán (CINEPY), "Estudio analítico de la situación económico y social de Yucatán," 1959, AGN, Fondo Banco Nacional de Crédito S. A. (Yucatán), Caja 2, exp. 1, p. 112.

125. CINEPY, "Estudio analítico," 111.

126. CINEPY, "Estudio analítico," 112, 120, 124–29.

127. AGN, Fondo Secretaría de Salubridad y Asistencia, Sección Comisión Constructora, Caja 72 (viejo), 355 (actual) , exp. 88, 151, 153, Caja 76 (viejo) 359 (actual); AGN, Fondo Secretaría de Salubridad y Asistencia, Sección Comisión Constructora, Vol. 91, expediente 39 (1960–64). At this time there were 15 Centers of Rural Health, located in Halacho, Muná, Opichén, Ixcan, Oxkatzcab, Sotuta, Mérida, Uca, X-Can, Motul, Pisto, Progreso, Sucilá, and Poblado Nuevo.

128. Bustamante, "La coordinación de los servicios sanitarios federales," 653.

Chapter 6

The Biomedicalization of Yucatán

Public health programs situated Yucatán in a complex nexus of local, national, and international relationships. One hundred years after the cholera epidemic of the 1850s coincided with the maturation of the biomedical project, which elites envisioned as a force to civilize and modernize the region. In constructing the biomedical community and public health infrastructure, Yucatec physicians utilized knowledge and technologies common to the Atlantic medical community. Late-nineteenth century medical knowledge sustained campaigns against diseases that could threaten the region's export economy. The project was handicapped—perhaps—by the social mentality of public health leaders, who lacked a commitment to combat the day-to-day illnesses that plagued most residents, especially in the countryside. By the 1960s, public health clinics operated in most Yucatec cities and towns, biomedical physicians had gained the exclusive authority of the state to practice medicine, and Yucatán's once autonomous medical system had become part of Mexico's medical bureaucracy. Biopower and state power were intrinsically linked.

The biomedicalization of Yucatán can be illustrated by the public health project in the interior of the state; in the epidemiologic disease transition; and by the location of Yucatec knowledge within the Atlantic medical community. Whites labeled the countryside as the "interior," the home of the Maya, who would be civilized by progress emanating from Mérida and Mexico City. As public health officials initiated activities in the interior, biomedical practices and "traditional" practices came into sharp juxtaposition, creating a system of medical pluralism. By the latter years of the twentieth century however, biomedicine had gained a dominant position, marginalizing once familiar practices and beliefs to the periphery of what is often referred to as "folk" medicine. The illnesses and diseases that troubled Yucatec residents changed dramatically as the region experienced an epidemiologic transition, in large part due to the biomedicalization project. Yucatec physicians participated actively in the medical community of the Atlantic World. Over time, their relative power diminished as specialized knowledge and technologies in the Atlantic "core" relegated the region to a medical "periphery." Yucatec "peripheralization" also coincided with the formation of the revolutionary state, a process that reduced Yucatán's power vis-à-vis the once-distant Mexico.

TRADITIONAL MEDICINE, MEDICAL PLURALISM, AND BIOMEDICALIZATION

Medical practices in Yucatán changed dramatically after the founding of the *Junta Superior de Sanidad* in 1894. At the beginning of the period, most people practiced what many anthropologists have labeled as "traditional" medicine, a remnant of the long colonial experience. Biomedicine was in its infancy, though it had a solid institutional foundation and firm political support in the Yucatec capital. The introduction of biomedicine in the countryside produced an era of medical pluralism—the coexistence of multiple medical systems—which gave way to a more complete biomedicalization by the end of the twentieth century.

Carnegie Institute anthropologists documented many dimensions of the spread of biomedicine into the Yucatec interior in the 1930s.[1] In *The Folk Culture of Yucatán*, Robert Redfield located the social development of communities along a cultural spectrum that ranged from "homogeneous" to "disorganized"; ideal types in the intellectual footsteps of Max Weber. The most "progressive" communities occupied the forefront of the spectrum, a conceptualization that saw the inevitable march of progress as eroding traditional society.[2] Alonso Villa Rojas exemplifies this "classic" anthropology in his observation that:

> The difference in the modes, customs, and dress between the Maya that lived in the henequen zone and those that remained in the periphery [of the corn zone] is now [1961] quite notable, in that the first group have been practically incorporated into the *campesino* class that is strongly connected to the city, while the others remained tied to the simple subsistence economy and the traditional norms of underdeveloped culture.[3]

Villa Rojas and others sought to reveal social differences in their community studies. Scholars associated with government agencies sought knowledge of indigenous medical practices in order to improve the efficacy of biomedical health systems, a pattern seen in the Andes and other regions.[4]

Yucatec scholar Eduardo Menéndez cautions against the casual use of the word "traditional" or "modern" in the region. Contact and colonization ended "authentic" Maya medicine; thereafter Yucatec medical practices were more a product of colonization than any pre-Columbian artifice. At the same time, the concept imposes a theoretical construct upon the study of historical processes and contemporary situations. The study of "traditional practices" produces "traditional" groups, a theoretical approach that negates the agency of historical actors. This locks social groups into ascribed positions defined by power relations, obscuring the dynamic and complex nature of Yucatec society. Menéndez equally rejects the label of "scientific medicine," preferring to focus upon the "conjuncture of practices used in different social contexts that reflects the values and norms of a particular society."[5] (This is akin to the "paradigm of meaning" implied in Press's concept of medical systems.) Following Menéndez, an account of the biomedicalization of interior Yucatán requires attention to social hierarchy and the role of medical institutions in structuring power relations and the development of new patterns of medicine.

In the Andes and many areas of Mesoamerica, medical pluralism emerged with the introduction of biomedicine by state officials or missionaries into indigenous or rural communities.[6] In Yucatán, public health officials and practitioners of biomedicine served as the most visible agents of medical change in the Yucatec interior; missionaries played a very limited role. A rich anthropological scholarship observed medical and social changes in a series of Yucatec communities, revealing the extension of biomedical practices into the countryside.

The campaign against smallpox constituted the initial biomedical experience for most people. Vaccinators acted sporadically through the nineteenth century, and then more systematically as the public health capacity of the state gained strength. Efforts to control yellow fever were concentrated in Mérida and Progreso, no doubt affecting Yucatec lives principally by a reduction of that disease. The development of the *Junta Superior* enabled widespread vaccination against the disease, dramatically reducing its occurrence in the early twentieth century. The development of auxiliary health units to fight the 1915 smallpox and the 1919 influenza epidemic created an initial institutional structure in larger towns in the interior, albeit with a concentration in the henequen zone.

Though Mérida dominated the biomedical infrastructure, private biomedical practitioners lived in more substantive towns such as Izamal, Peto, and Tizimín. Both the 1924 directory of physicians and a 1932 report indicated that upwards of twenty-five percent of all biomedical doctors lived outside the capital.[7] These physicians often served on the auxiliary health boards, and facilitated the expansion of biomedicine into the countryside. Pharmacists or lay practitioners—whom the titled doctors often labeled as charlatans—supplemented their activities. Menéndez suggests that private physicians, vendors of patent medicines, and itinerant healers affected the lives of rural dwellers far more than did the activities of public health workers.[8] Redfield observed in the 1930s that residents of Chan Kom lacked access to public health officials, but that they regularly visited the Carnegie sponsored clinic at Chichen Itza, sought out itinerant healers, and utilized the local pharmacy for biomedical supplies. At the same time, they made regular use of "traditional" medicine and healers.[9]

Beginning in the 1930s, state and federal officials extended public health care to many areas of the henequen and corn zones. The social assistance program of the *Henequeneros de Yucatán* quickly developed a hierarchy of facilities offering periodic services in small communities, permanent service in towns, and hospital care in Mérida. By the early 1950s, over a third of Yucatán's citizens had access to ASHOY facilities. Federal efforts in the corn zone were less ambitious, with four Centers of Rural Hygiene in place by 1937.[10]

State and federal officials agreed that more facilities were needed in the corn zone, but the region's *ejidos* lacked the capacity to pay for services. Dr. Arturo Erosa Barbachano reported to the second Yucatec Medical Congress in 1944 that the limited numbers of Rural Hygiene Clinics left most *campesinos* with the choice of traveling to the Hospital O'Horan in Mérida, seeking relief from nonprofessional healers, or remaining untreated. Most, he claimed, preferred not to go to Mérida, leaving him to support the creation of a system of rural hospitals.[11] Governor José González Beytia reported in 1949 that the ASHOY had begun to expand services in the corn zone. *Campesinos* in Muná, Sotuta, Sucilá, and Cenotillo would be served through ASHOY clinics, with an emphasis on primary care and maternity services.[12] In addition to health care objectives, officials sought to extend the authority of biomedicine "to protect these communities from the actions of midwives, empirics and *curanderos*."[13]

The construction of rural hospitals dovetailed with the need to diversify Yucatán's agricultural base. Henequen had weakened the regional economy, a domination that planners in the 1950s thought could be reduced by increased corn production, cattle grazing, fruit trees, and sugar cane. This at least was the hope of the National Commission on Irrigation, which sought to take advantage of the fertility of the corn zone to diversify agricultural production. Erosa Barbachano suggested that the construction of rural hospitals in towns such as Tizimín, Valladolid, Peto, and Ticul would complement the irrigation projects aimed at supporting the development of citrus or other crops bound for the urban market. Ticul, for example, was located at the juncture of multiple rail lines, and would offer access to health care for more than 33,000 people. It would also serve the 400 employees of the irrigation commission, who also lacked access to health care.[14]

Federal programs directed toward indigenous peoples aggressively advanced the biomedical project. These began early in the Revolution and matured in the National Indigenist Institute (1948). The INI created "penetration roads" into indigenous regions, bringing isolated places of "refuge" into the "civilized" national framework. These "penetration roads" facilitated the gradual erosion of traditional medicine, leading to the acceptance of biomedicine, and creating reliance upon the new state structures.[15] INI officials pursued a strategy of lowering "scientific medicine to the communities' cultural level," so as to avoid immediate rejection. Critical factors in their success included respect for residents and their culture, a capacity to speak the local language, creating penetration roads that brought state power into indigenous sectors. Gonzalo Aguirre Beltrán insisted that local INI officials "become part of the community," and slowly develop trusting relations.[16] For June Nash, the INI constituted a hegemonic effort to assert control over indigenous people, albeit one that gave local communities certain latitudes over which programs might be instituted in their communities.[17] Though an INI program was not begun until 1958 in Yucatán, the 1956 Rural Wellbeing program adhered to similar methods and objectives.

The penetration roads of the INI connected indigenous communities to the nation, serving as an insightful metaphor for state formation. Public health programs facilitated the penetration of biomedicine into indigenous communities, catalyzing relationships between local actors and state agents that gradually displaced traditional medicine. Medical students fulfilling their social service obligation in indigenous communities were cautioned not to reject local *curanderos*, but to establish an atmosphere of trust with local residents. An official pamphlet noted that most *curandero* activities were not dangerous; and that their "psychotherapeutic" value should not be discounted. As trust was established, physicians would be sought out more frequently, especially among the younger generations.[18]

Whether from public or private initiatives, by the late 1960s, biomedicine had become an accepted part of the rural Yucatec healing profile. Press describes how public health agencies were important medical fixtures in the corn zone, helping to inculcate biomedical beliefs at the community level.[19] Most residents seemingly accepted biomedical practices as complementary to *curanderismo*. As Redfield related, "perhaps it is nearer the truth to say that no definite choice between old and new remedy is made. Rather, the new is added to the old. If one does not work, the other is tried."[20] Generational differences characterized the acceptance of new practices, as residents under the age of thirty tended to rely upon biomedicine because of its recognized efficacy and perceived social prestige, while older members of the community adhered to traditional healing patterns.[21] Ruth Gubler noted that in late-twentieth century Yucatán few young people appeared to be interested in traditional healers.[22]

Biomedicine came to dominate the state. By the last decades of the twentieth century, most communities had a medical clinic associated with the Mexican or Yucatec governments, a pharmacy stocked with biomedical materials, and a private biomedical practitioner. Once attempts at household cures had failed, these would be the healers of first choice. Herbs would be sold in the local marketplace, and the medicinal value of plants was commonly known. Traditional approaches increasingly occupied marginal positions within the medical system of the region.

PUBLIC HEALTH AND THE EPIDEMIOLOGIC TRANSITION

Healing practices mediate the relationships between diseases and human bodies. In the years after contact, Yucatec healers likely had little capacity to affect the "natural" course of diseases. Spaniards brought smallpox, typhoid fever, measles, and other contagions that led to a dramatic population loss in Yucatán, diseases that indigenous healers appeared unable to cure. The appearance of yellow fever in the mid-1600s afflicted native and *dzule* alike; forcing colonial authorities to undertake limited public health activities, actions that regrettably had little impact on the course of the disease. Epidemics of the day might be slowed by quarantine, but prayer and supplication seemed equally effective—or futile. A slowly developed resistance to crowd diseases enabled indigenous populations to increase after the mid-1700s, interrupted only by the mid-nineteenth-century Caste Wars. The nineteenth-century anti-smallpox campaign demonstrated the ability to control the spread of a disease, even while institutional capacity and political antipathies hindered its efficacy. As smallpox and yellow fever became endemic to the region, they periodically erupted into minor epidemics that plagued native and white alike, but without the dread of the early colonial period. Germ theory spurred the development of vaccines to reduce the impact of diphtheria, anthrax, typhoid, and numerous other diseases. By the mid-twentieth century, morbidity rates were dominated by gastrointestinal and chronic diseases, as contagions caused a decreasing number of illnesses.

This historical process parallels Omran's epidemiologic theory and raises questions about the impact of Yucatec public health agencies upon the disease environment.[23] Omran hypothesized that differing mortality rates corresponded to "ages" dominated by distinct patterns of disease. These ages are seen in demographic and morbidity patterns. Initially, mortality rates fluctuate dramatically due to epidemic contagions and frequent famines, an age comparable to the impact of conquest on native peoples. Yucatán's eighteenth-century demographic recovery of the region matches Omran's "age of receding pandemics," though the Caste War negatively impacted the pace of demographic expansion. Omran next envisions an "Age of Degenerative and Man-Made Diseases," an epidemiologic transition when epidemic diseases are brought under control, standards of living and hygiene improve, and when "medical and public health factors come into play" as factors in mortality reduction. Different areas of the world experienced the final transition at different times (the accelerated, contemporary, and delayed models), largely due to their stages of economic development and health care effects upon mortality rates.[24] Though in some ways a blunt demographic measurement reflective of a modernization ideological lens, the final demographic increase is clearly visible in Yucatán after the 1960s, fitting within Omran's "delayed" model.[25]

Death rates began to decline in Mexico and Latin America in the late nineteenth century, first in urban and then in rural regions. Birth rates, by contrast, did not begin to decline until the 1960s, marking an epidemiological transition and rapid population expansion.[26] To what extent did public health agencies change the disease profile of Yucatán? How did public health activities facilitate the epidemiologic transition in the first half of the twentieth century?

Limited data complicate an answer to these fundamental questions. Mortality data prior to the 1920s is extremely limited, and the categorization of diseases varied enormously. Data exists for Mérida for 1905, the

Figure 6.1 Population Trends, 1900–1995

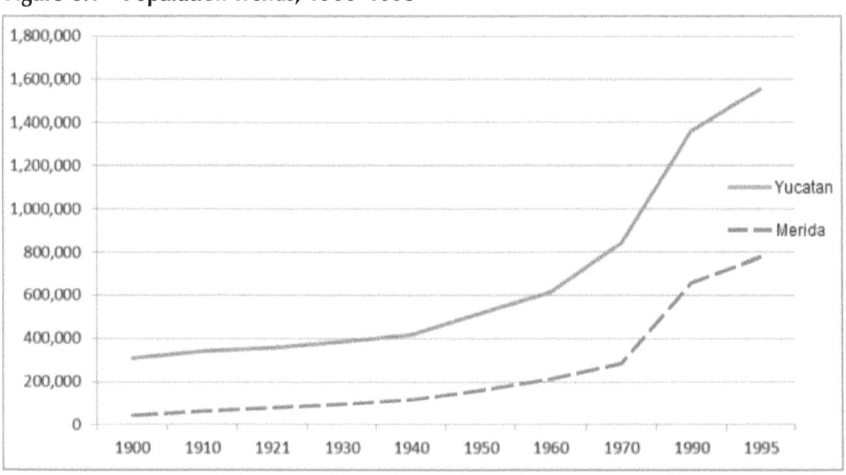

Source: Sherburne F. Cook and Woodrow Wilson Borah, "Population of Yucatán," in Essays in Population History: Mexico and the Caribbean, Volume 2 (Berkeley: University of California Press, 1974).

early 1930s, and the late 1940s. Statewide data exist for the mid-1940s, late 1950s, and more consistently thereafter. Federal officials published standardized mortality and morbidity information during the last third of the century. Other information describes health conditions in rural communities at various times. Data for Mérida in July–September 1904 indicate, for example, that half of the 3,433 deaths were of children less than two years old, 799 from gastrointestinal diseases.[27] Though data such as this must be used with caution, deaths from smallpox, yellow fever, and malaria had declined markedly by the 1920s.[28] Gastrointestinal diseases caused the largest number of deaths in both urban and rural settings through most of the twentieth century (see Tables 6.1, 6.2, and 6.3.)

Classification of diseases complicates data analysis. Gastrointestinal labels likely captured a range of maladies. In its survey of diseases in the 1920s, the Carnegie report suggests that dysentery, gastro-enteritis, enteritis, colitis,

Table 6.1 Comparative Mortality Rates, Mérida

	1905	*1944–48*
Gastrointestinal	32.41%	21%
Tuberculosis	10.6%	2.2%
Heart diseases	2.9%	3.1%
Pneumonia	2.4%	5.6%
Bronchitis	2.3%	5.0%
Senility	2.2%	6.6%
Malaria	2.2%	5.0%
Dysentery	2.0%	2.9%
Malignant tumors	1.4%	1.7%
Influenza	.8%	1.5%

Sources: La Revista Médica de Yucatán, July 1906; Tomás Marentes Miranda, *Reseña histórica, geográfica y estadísticas del Estado de Yucatán* (México: NP, 1951), appendix.

Table 6.2 Statewide Mortality Rates, 1940–60 (rates per 100,000)

Diseases	*1940*	*1950*	*1960*
Infectious and Parasitical	1253	740	525
Respiratory	305	175	152
Unclear cause	212	152	177
Perinatal	118	102	107
Circulatory	90	100	95
Digestive	85	70	95
Nutritional	82		46
Nervous System	60	41	20
Tumors	32	49	58
Urinary	29	17	10

Source: Menéndez, *Poder, estratificación y salud,* 179. He compiles this table from the Federal Bureau of Statistics.

Table 6.3 Mortality Rates, 1965 (rates per 100,000 deaths)

	Yucatán	*Mérida*
Gastro-intestinal Diseases	140.8	132.3
Influenza and Phenomena	94.6	146.8
Perinatal Illnesses	83.2	49.9
Bronchitis	66.7	25.7
Heart-Related Diseases	58.0	62.8
Malignant Tumors	42.4	35.0
Nutritional Deficiencies	32.2	14.3
Cerebrovascular Illnesses	30.4	
Measles	26.1	14.2
Cirrhosis of the liver	25.8	21.1

Source: "Datos relativos a la salud pública en el estado de Yucatán, 1971," AGN, Fondo SSA, Sección Dirección General de Servicios Coordinados de Salud Pública en los Estados y Territorios, Vol. 39 (viejo), 589 (actual).

and even typhoid fever might be included in the broad category of "gastro-intestinal diseases."[29] Menéndez groups similar illnesses into an "infectious and parasitical diseases" category.[30] Granting variations in disease categorization, mortality and morbidity rates from gastrointestinal illnesses appear to have fallen slowly in both Mérida and in rural settings over the course of the twentieth century.

Commentators unanimously agreed that Yucatán's poor water quality contributed to high rates of gastrointestinal disease. They differed—to a degree—on what could be done to address the problem. In the 1940s, physicians José F. Diaz and Benjamín Góngora Triay suggested that 80 percent of Mérida's residents used rainwater stored in cisterns or *aljibes*. Others used well water drawn from the aquifer, the same source as the Mérida Yucatán Water Company. The limestone soil allowed sewage to pollute the aquifer, which was especially problematic early in the rainy season. While the Water Company purified the water, most residents did not. Only five percent of Mérida's 23,437 houses had sanitary sewer conditions. Most relied upon cesspools or simply used the soil in their yards.[31] Díaz and Góngora argued that contamination of Mérida's aquifer constituted "the most serious sanitary problem of the city."[32] Rural communities were comparably slow in gaining access to potable water, with the vast majority using traditional sources well past the mid-century. (See Table 5.1) Askinasy and Menéndez acknowledge that the lack of potable water lay at the root of the problem, but that socio-economic conditions in the countryside were equally culpable.[33]

High rates of gastrointestinal diseases led to the death of one in three infants during their first year of life.[34] In the late 1930s, Rafael Ramos Galván, head of Yucatán's *Servicio de Asistencia Infantil* (Infant Assistance Program), conducted a study of Mérida's infant mortality rates and suggested

Table 6.4 Morbidity, 1945, Yucatán Henequen Social Assistance Facilities

Intestinal Parasites	33.1%
Illnesses of the Digestive System	30.8%
Respiratory Illnesses	19.3%
Malaria	7.1%
Urinary Illnesses	4.8%
Syphilis	2.6%
Tuberculosis	1.5%
Typhoid Fever	.7%

Source: La Revista Médica de Yucatán, August 31, 1946. The data are drawn from ASHOY facilities, the Hospital O'Horán, the Hospital del Niño, and the Hernández Fajardo and Peniche Cantón laboratories.

Table 6.5 Community Access to Potable Water, 1971

Residents	*Communities*	*Number and % without potable water*
1–500	2182	2170–95%
500–2499	141	106–75%
2500+	38	27–76%

Source: "Datos relativos a la salud pública en el Estado de Yucatán, 1971."

that two-thirds of these deaths were from gastrointestinal diseases.[35] (Please see Table 6.4.) A few years later, officials with the social assistance program of the HOY estimated that fully ninety percent of all children in the henequen zone suffered from some form of intestinal parasite.[36] Askinasy suspected that infant mortality rates were somewhat higher in the countryside than in the city, and that perhaps half of all deaths in rural sector took place before the age of five,[37] an observation confirmed by data from the corn zone and the capital.[38] Public health officials commented at the 1941 opening of the Children's Hospital that "the diet of the Maya people has led to a weakening of the race and, as a result, an alarming coefficient of infant mortality."[39]

Sanitary officials did little to rectify poor water quality. Urban officials had made inspections of sewage and water facilities as part of their yellow fever and malaria campaigns, but Díaz and Góngora complained the inspections were rare and cursory—and limited to the capital city. Potable water was clearly the remedy to waterborne disease but, until that was available, educational campaigns leading to changed patterns of personal hygiene were necessary.[40] ASHOY officials urged the use of chlorine at community wells on henequen *ejidos*, the development and utilization of sanitary latrines, and hygienic education. Murals, leaflets, and films in Maya would form the foundation of public education recognition of the limited use of Spanish in many areas of the interior.[41] Infant mortality rates in the corn zone fell steadily after 1940, perhaps in response to these measures. Menéndez suggests that access to medications and private doctors played an important role, as did decreased

Table 6.6 Infant Mortality, Mérida, 1927–36

1927	*1928*	*1929*	*1930*	*1931*	*1932*	*1933*	*1934*	*1935*	*1936*
36.6	30.3	29	35.9	31	30	30.6	26.3	36.5	27.6

Source: Diaz and Góngora, "La higiene," 403.

Table 6.7 Infant Mortality, Corn Region, 1940–1990 (per 1,000 births)

1940	180.5
1950	143.4
1960	103.0
1970	97.4
1980	80.9
1990	34.7

Source: Gurri, Balam Pereira, and Moran, "Well-Being Changes," 594.

labor demands as henequen estates became community property and as the profitability of this export declined.[42]

The epidemiologic transition appears to have taken place by the 1970s. Actions by public health officials led to a general improvement in Yucatán's disease environment prior to the 1950s, primarily due to the construction of public health infrastructure in much of the state. In 1964, for example, *Centros Primarios Materno Infantiles* operated in nineteen smaller towns in the corn zone of the state.[43] Major public health initiatives included vaccination programs against diphtheria, whooping cough, tetanus, polio, and measles, coupled with the elimination of malaria through the use of DDT. The generalized use of pharmaceuticals, inoculation campaigns of the 1960s and 1970s accelerated the transition, facilitated by the activities of private physicians in small towns. Gurri, Pereira, and Moran note that regional "integration into the state" sustained the epidemiological transition in the early 1970s. Integration came by way of public health intervention and an increased availability of salaried labor positions. By the 1990s, residents had near-universal access to biomedical health care at public and private facilities, potable water, and electricity. Sanitary and vaccination programs in the 1970s served as a potent catalyst for lowered infant mortality rates. Greater declines came from a "steady improvement in living conditions" and correlated with circular migration to and from Mérida and changes in agricultural production.[44] Few, Mercado, Graizbord, and Albornoz Mendoza date the transition to the same period, marked especially by the decline of deaths from gastrointestinal diseases.[45]

These data suggest that the epidemiologic transition occurred in the context of the broad process of biomedicalization. Public health programs, especially childhood vaccination campaigns, constituted the foundation for the transformation of the disease environment. State and federal health officials combined to construct a public health infrastructure that served the overwhelming majority of Yucatec residents. The pharmaceutical revolution and the changing nature of the region's political economy complemented and strengthened those efforts. At the end of the twentieth century, a different range of diseases afflicted residents of Yucatán than had one hundred years earlier, leading to a significantly healthier population, albeit one with more chronic illnesses.

YUCATÁN AND THE ATLANTIC MEDICAL COMMUNITY

Biomedicine became the dominant approach to healing within the Atlantic region over the course of the twentieth century. Power associated with biomedicine has often been envisioned as flowing from a western European/US core into Latin American and African peripheries through direct colonialism, institutions of higher education, or medical associations. Studies of tropical medicine fit within this perspective, seeing medicine as a tool of imperialist projects.[46] By contrast, other scholarship characterizes the "interaction of experts from different countries and the transnational movements of materials and people as an intrinsic part of biomedical knowledge production."[47] While medical knowledge or technology might originate in England, France, or Germany, physicians and research groups in Brazil, Colombia, Cuba, and Argentina would utilize scientific understandings in support of national objectives.

The ebb and flow of economic and political forces altered the positions of the Yucatec public health system within the Atlantic medical community. Henequen wealth and easily accessible medical knowledge sustained the creation of an extensive public health system in the early years of the twentieth century. Sources of knowledge, medical education, and medical journals demonstrate Yucatec physician's participation in the biomedical community, with no dominant source for the medical knowledge evident in the peninsula.[48] Yucatec priorities dictated the course of public health activities, not the priorities of central Mexico or international agents. Over time, however, external forces exerted increasing power and influence in the state. By the mid-twentieth century, Yucatán occupied a decided peripheral position, as the revolutionary Mexican state gained strength, and as biomedical technologies and practices became increasingly complex and less accessible.

Late nineteenth-century Yucatec organizations appear to have been less subject to foreign influences than Mexico City's *Consejo de Salubridad*. Paul Ross argues that international, and especially French, medical ideas shaped the mentalities and actions of physicians associated with public health in the national capital prior to the 1880s. Many physicians traveled to Europe for both conferences and advanced training, and returned home to use those understandings in the Mexican capital.[49] Marcos Cueto and Steven Palmer see the potent French influence throughout Latin America.[50] By contrast, most

Yucatec officials who formed the *Sociedad Médico-Farmaceutica* (1871) and the *Junta Superior de Sanidad* (1894) acquired their education in Mérida. All but two of the thirteen physician members of the Medical-Pharmaceutical Society studied at the School of Medicine in Yucatán; one trained first in Mérida before additional training in Paris; another trained first in New York and then Paris.[51] All of the seven original officers of the *Junta Superior* graduated from Mérida's School of Medicine.[52]

Foreign education among Yucatec physicians was more common in the nineteenth than twentieth century, and no single country dominated external education. Slightly over one-fourth of the physicians titled by the school between 1820 and 1890 were educated abroad; of the 53 doctors, eleven graduated from Cuban universities, ten from schools in the USA, five from France, and four apiece from Mexico City and Spain. The number of physicians educated abroad declined to 15 percent between 1890 and 1933.[53] Still, even these limited numbers indicate an active membership in the Atlantic medical community, as did the consumption of knowledge and technological evidenced in journals and associations.

Public health agencies drew deeply upon Atlantic medical knowledge. Writers for *La Emulación* in the 1870s spoke of the need to institutionalize public health, citing French and German use—for example—of medical statistics to monitor disease. The *Boletín de Higiene*, the mouthpiece of the *Junta Superior de Sanidad*, spoke proudly of public health as the "foundation for wealth and social well-being," noting that the organization followed in the footsteps of French, English, and German public health pioneers.[54] The medical press associated with the *Junta Superior* regularly drew upon European sources for their articles on tuberculosis,[55] diphtheria,[56] slaughterhouses,[57] or dysentery.[58] In 1911, for example, Rafael Betancourt urged that the *Junta* approach the governor to create a commission to address high rates of infant mortality, a commission that he hoped would draw upon methods from Cuba and Uruguay.[59] A similar proposal twelve years later suggested United States "Healthy Infant Brigades" as appropriate for Yucatán.[60]

From its establishment in 1905 as the mouthpiece of the Yucatec Medical Society, *La Revista Médica de Yucatán* illuminates the international nature of medical knowledge and its movement through the Atlantic medical community. The paper generally opened its pages with local studies, then reprinted articles from the international medical press, and closed with notes from medical associations. These patterns are clear in snapshots from the *Yucatec Medical Review* from 1918, 1940, and 1950. In 1918, Ricardo Sauri writes about swelling of the eyes, a study with Spanish intellectual foundations; Carrillo Gil discusses childhood nutritional problems in 1940; as did Tomas Peniche Alvarez ten years later. Translations from the international press might come from Havana (*La Crónica Médico-Quirúgica* in 1918); Buenos

Aires (*El Dia Médica* in 1940); or London (British Medical Information Service in 1950). No country served as the predominant source of articles, though Spanish language sources appear more frequently than translated studies. The *Revista* usually concluded its issues with notes on the exchange of medical publications from abroad. In 1940, 54 publications were received, 17 from Mexico, five from the United States, 20 from Latin America, 10 from Europe, and one from Japan.[61]

Diseases such as yellow fever, cholera, and malaria linked Yucatec physicians to the international medical community, especially through the International Health Board of the Rockefeller Foundation. In many countries the IHB played a significant role in structuring public health programs, though not in Yucatán. The IHB campaign of the 1920s enhanced existing antimalaria efforts, especially as federal sanitary delegates increased their influence in the states, but did little to alter the public health landscape of the region. By contrast, Cuba occupied a special place in Yucatán's medical community. A Cuban physician introduced homeopathy to the region, and Yucatec physicians drew deeply upon Cuban knowledge in response to the cholera epidemic in the 1850s.[62] The knowledge/technologies of yellow fever prevention came from Cuba to Yucatán directly, as well as through the 1903 federal campaign against the disease.[63] Cuban-born physician Eduardo Urzaiz Rodríguez headed the Asilo Ayala for 24 years, and many other physicians were members of Cuban medical organizations or migrated from the island.

The growth in the international pharmaceutical community was the most noticeable change in the pages of *La Revista Médica de Yucatán* over its fifty-year history (1905–1955). At the start of the century, most drugs appear to have been mixed from raw materials by physicians or pharmacists. Advertisements were limited, with chemicals, instruments, and services of physicians most common. Beginning in the 1920s, advertisements in the newsletter reveal the emergence of the vast biomedical pharmaceutical industry. Bayer, Eli Lilly and Company, Schering-Kahlbaum AG, Ebrey Chemical Works, and Park Davis and Company were among the many international firms offering their wares for sale. By 1950, the paper advertised various drugs from Casa Bayer; Switzerland's Wander Company; J. Boulard's antiseptic; "Sulfamargina" pills from Garcol: Laboratorios Lauzier; Milo drink from Nestlé; and Paris's Roussel Group. In the 1920s, most of the drugs appear to have been imported; by 1950 most were made in Mexico City by international companies and marketed within the nation.[64] The commercialization of biomedicine in the first half of the twentieth century transformed Yucatec physicians from producers into consumers. This increased importance of pharmaceuticals originating in medical centers was no doubt common in other areas of the Atlantic medical community.

The most visible process of peripheralization involves the relationship between the state of Yucatán and the Mexican government. Wealth from henequen sustained the construction of a Yucatec public health system that was in legal and practical terms nearly autonomous from the federal government. The growth of the revolutionary state slowly changed that relationship, even as Yucatec public health officials capitalized on the nationalization of henequen plantations to construct the massive social assistance program of the *Henequeneros de Yucatán*. The *Secretaría de Salubridad y Asistencia* (SSA), authorized in 1943, established an institutional frame for federal-directed public health, a culmination of years of effort to subordinate Yucatec public health activities to the Mexican nation. When henequen prices collapsed after World War II, and the *Henequeneros de Yucatán* was forced to dissolve, the SSA assumed control of its public health network. Yucatec-directed public health organizations persisted, but over time most were subsumed into the national orbit.[65]

Yucatec public health officials worked within a complex Atlantic biomedical community. Despite the multi-nodal nature of Atlantic medical communities, biomedical power tended toward asymmetrical relations, whether seen from broad international or from intra-national perspectives. Centers and peripheries remained as valuable conceptualizations of the flows of knowledge and power. Relations between centers and peripheries were dynamic, with medical knowledge, technologies, and power within the Atlantic biomedical community "flatter" in the nineteenth century and more "centered" over time. Henequen wealth enabled Yucatec officials to construct a public health system that differed little in practice, ideology, or purpose from similar organizations in Mexico City, Buenos Aires, Salvador de Bahia, or other cities,[66] though resources and its relationship to the national government individualized its history. This constitutes the "rupture" that illustrates the perceived utility of science by the Yucatec intellegenia,[67] even though the Yucatec medical and scientific communities would be subsumed into larger national and international power structures.

Over the course of the twentieth century, medical specialization, techniques, and technologies slowly created greater distinctions within the Atlantic medical community, with clear loci of authority and influence. The Mexican Revolution spawned the reconceptualization of state functions that led to federal expansion into Yucatec health affairs in the 1930s. After World War II, strengthening revolutionary public health initiatives coincided with the collapse of henequen prices, facilitating the nationalization of much of the Yucatec public health system in the 1950s. By mid-century, Yucatec public health practitiners had become subordinate to the Mexican state and increasingly reliant upon the technologies and knowledge of centers of biomedicine and international public health. Amid this slow process of peripheralization, Yucatec physicians continued their membership in the Atlantic medical community, drawing upon it for knowledge, technologies, and training.

Changing power dynamics infused these relationships. The henequen boom underpinned the establishment and growth of the *Junta Superior de Sanidad* and the emergence of the region as an economic powerhouse. Yucatec elite resisted efforts by the revolutionary federal government in the 1910s and 1920s to control the henequen industry, and forced Cárdenas to modify plans for the nationalization of henequen estates. The social assistance program of the *Henequeneros de Yucatán* led to the rapid expansion of public health facilities in the henequen zone, institutions matched by the federal government in the corn zone. The post–World War II decline in henequen prices led to the federal takeover of the "Gran Ejido" and its health facilities in 1955. Without the wealth that had sustained Yucatec autonomy in public health decision-making, Yucatán reverted to the status of a marginalized, poorer Mexican state. The government created by the revolutionary process would assume public health leadership in the second half of the twentieth century, furthering the biomedicalization of the peninsula.

NOTES

1. The National Geographic magazine consistently projects this image. Peter Hervik, "The Mysterious Maya of National Geographic," *Journal of Latin American Anthropology* 4:1 (September 1998), 166–197. See also Catherine A. Lutz and Jane L. Collins, *Reading National Geographic* (Chicago: University of Chicago Press, 1993).

2. Redfield, *The Folk Culture of Yucatán* (Chicago: University of Chicago Press, 1941); Redfield, *A Village that Chose Progress: Chan Kom Revisited* (Chicago: University of Chicago Press, 1962).

3. Villa Rojas, *Los mayas de las tierras Bajas* (México: INAH (Instituto Nacional de Antropología e Historia) CAPFCE, SEP (Secretaría de Educación Pública), 1961, 35.

4. Ann Miles and Thomas Leatherman, "Perspectives on Medical Anthropology in the Andes," in Joan D. Koss-Chioino, Thomas Leatherman, and Christine Greenway, *Medical Pluralism in the Andes* (New York: Routledge, 2003), 3–15; Walter Randolph Adams and John P. Hawkins, *Health Care in Guatemala: Confronting Medical Pluralism in a Developing Country* (Norman: University of Oklahoma Press, 2007); Carlos Viesca Treviño, "*Curanderismo* in Mexico and Guatemala: Its Historical Evolution from the Sixteenth to the Nineteenth Century," in *Mesoamerican Healers*, ed. by Brad R. Huber and Alan R. Sandstrom (Austin: Texas University Press, 2001), 47–65.

5. Eduardo L. Menéndez, "Medicina tradicional, atención primaria y la problematica del alcholismo," in *Medicina tradicional y atención primaria: Ensayos en*

homenaje a Gonzalo Aquirre Beltran (México: Cuadernos de la Casa Chata, No. 159, 1987), 27–32.

6. A classic account is Libbet Crandon-Malamud, *From the Fat of Our Souls: Social Change, Political Processes, and Medical Pluralism in Bolivia* (Berkeley: University of California Press, 1991).

7. *La Revista Médica de Yucatán*, March 1924; Junta Superior de Sanidad to Governor, January 30, 1931, Mérida, AGEY, FPE, Sección JSS, Serie Copiador de Oficios, Volume 149, entry 89.

8. Menéndez, *Poder, estratificación y salud,* 212, 451–55.

9. Redfield, *Chan Kom: A Maya Village*, 171.

10. Departamento de Salubridad Pública, Directorio General, *La Oficina Central de Higiene Rural y Servicios Coordinados en los estados* (Mexico: Talleres del Imprenta del Departamento de Salubridad Pública, 1937), 64, 69.

11. Arturo Erosa Barbachano, "Necesidad de pequeños hospitales rurales," in *Memorias del segundo congreso médico peninsular* (Mérida: Díaz Massa, 1945), 266.

12. *Informe del Ciudadano Profesor José Gutiérrez Beytia, Gobernador Constitucional del Estado, año de 1948* (Mérida: Gobierno del Estado de Yucatán, 1949), 80–81.

13. *Informe del Ciudadano Profesor José Gutiérrez Beytia, Gobernador Constitucional del Estado, año de 1948*, 81.

14. Erosa Barbachano, "Necesidad de pequeños hospitales rurales," 267.

15. Stephen E. Lewis, "Mexico's National Indigenist Institute and the Negotiation of Applied Anthropology in Highland Chiapas, 1951–1954," *Ethnohistory* 55:4 (Fall 2008), 617.

16. Gonzalo Aguirre Beltrán, *Programas de salud en la situación intercultural* (México DF: INI, 1955), 12, 19.

17. June C. Nash, *Maya Visions: The Quest for Autonomy in an Age of Globalization* (New York: Routledge, 2001), 66–67, 133.

18. Luis Alberto Vargas, ed., ¿Que *debo saber sobre medicina tradicional durante mi servicio social?* (México: Editorial del Semenario la Medicina del Hombre en su totalidad, 1981).

19. Irwin Press, *Tradition and Adaptation: Life in a Modern Yucatán Maya Village* (Westport, CT: Greenwood Press, 1975).

20. Redfield, *Chan Kom Revisited*, 130.

21. Robert Charles Harman, *Cambios médicos y sociales en una comunidad maya-tzeltal* (México: Instituto Nacional Indigenista y Secretaría de Educación Pública, 1974); Denise F. Brown, "Life in the Fast Lane: Change over three Generations in a Yucatec Maya Town," in *Maya Survivalism. Acta Mesoamericana* Vol. 12 (Verlag: Anton Saurwein, 2001), 217–23.

22. Ruth Gubler, "*La medicine tradicional en Yucatán a través de los siglos*," in Ruth Gubler, organizer and compiler, *Yucatán a través de los siglos* (Memorias del 49th Congreso Internacional de Americanistas, Quito, Ecuador, 1997) (Mérida: Universidad Autónoma de Yucatán, 2001), 229–47.

23. Abdel R. Omran, "The Epidemiologic Transition: A Theory of the Epidemiology of Population Change," *The Milbank Memorial Fund Quarterly* 49:4 (1971),

509–38. Many scholars have utilized Omran's theory, sparking a vast and sophisticated literature. See, for example, George Weisz and Jesse Olsyzkno-Gryn, "The Theory of Epidemiologic Transition: The Origins of a Citation Classic," *Journal of the History of Medicine and the Allied Sciences* 65:3 (July 2010), 287–326; Graziella Caselli, France Meslé, and Jacques Vallin, "Epidemiologic Transition Theory Exceptions," *Genus* 58:1 (January-March 2002), 9–51.

24. Omran, "The Epidemiologic Transition."

25. Omran, "The Epidemiologic Transition," 754.

26. Jorge Brea, "Population Dynamics in Latin America," *Population Bulletin* 58:1 (March 2003), 11.

27. *Boletín de Estadística*, July 1, 1905.

28. Menéndez, *Poder, estratificación y salud*, 164–166.

29. Shattuck, *The Peninsula of Yucatán*, 361.

30. Menéndez, *Poder, estratificación y salud*, 178.

31. José F. Díaz and Benjamín Gongora Triay, "La higiene," in *Enciclopedia Yucatanese*. 2nd ed. (Mérida: Edición Oficial del Gobierno de Yucatán, 1977), Tomo VI, 382–84.

32. Díaz and Góngora Triay, "La higiene," 383.

33. Askinay, *El problema agrario*, 21.

34. Shattuck, *The Peninsula of Yucatán*, 396–98.

35. Diaz and Góngora Triay, "La higiene," 401.

36. *La Revista Médica de Yucatán*, August 31, 1946.

37. Askinasy, *El problema agrario*, 23–24.

38. Francisco D. Gurri, Gilberto Balam Pereira, Emilio F. Moran, "Well-Being Changes in Response to 30 Years of Regional Integration in Maya Populations from Yucatán, Mexico," *American Journal of Human Biology* 15 (2001), 594.

39. *El Hospital del Niño* (Mérida: Gobierno del Estado de Yucatán, 1940), 10.

40. Diaz and Góngora, "La higiene," 393.

41. *La Revista Médica de Yucatán*, August 31, 1946.

42. Menéndez, *Poder, estratificación y salud,* 212, 249, 451.

43. AGN, FSSA, Sec. Comissión Constructora, Caja 76 (viejo)/ 359 (actual).

44. Gurri, Balam Pereira, and Moran, "Well-Being Changes," 592, 596, 597, 600; Menéndez, *Poder, estratificación y salud,* 261.

45. Roger Few, Alfonso Mercado, Boris Graizbord, Lilian Albornoz Mendoza, "Climatic Hazards, Health Risk and Response, Case Study 4: Yucatán, Mexico," UK Economic and Research Council, January 2008, 10.

46. As an example, see Alexandra Minna Stern, "Yellow Fever Crusade: US Colonialism, Tropical Medicine, and the International Politics of Mosquito Control, 1900–1920," in *Disease, Globalization and Security, 1850 to the Present*, ed. by Alison Bashford (London: Palgrave MacMillan, 2006), 41–59.

47. Anne-Emanuel Birn and Raúl Neochochea López, "Footprints on the Future: Looking Forward to the History of Health and Medicine in the Twenty-First Century," *Hispanic American Historical Review* 91:3 (August 2011), 523.

48. *La Emulación* (La Sociedad Médico-Farmacéutica, 1873–79); *La Higiene* (Consejo Superior de Salubridad del Estado de Yucatán, 1895); *La Revista Médica de*

Yucatán (Sociedad Médica Yucateca, 1905–1953); *La Higiene* (Dirección General de Salubridad e Higiene 1918–1919); *Revista de Medicina Homeopática* (1921); *Boletín Mensual del Sindicato de Médicos y Profesionistas Conexos de Yucatán* (mid-1930s); *Asistencia Social* (late 1940s, associated with the social assistance program of the *Henequeneros de Yucatán*).

49. Paul Ross, "Mexico's Superior Health Council and the American Public Health Association: The Transnational Archive of Porfirian Public Health, 1887–1910," *Hispanic American Historical Review* 89:4 (November 2009), 574–76.

50. Marcos Cueto and Steven Palmer, *Medicine and Public Health in Latin America: A History* (New York: Cambridge University Press, 2014).

51. *La Emulación*, January 1873, May 1874.

52. *Boletín de Higiene*, May 5, 1895.

53. *La Revista de Mérida*, 17:12 (1934), 532–34.

54. *Boletín de Higiene*, May 5, 1895.

55. *La Crónica Médica de Yucatán*, January 31, 1891.

56. *Boletín de Higiene*, May 5, 1895.

57. *La Revista Médica de Yucatán*, December 1908.

58. *La Revista Médica de Yucatán*, July 1909.

59. *La Revista Médica de Yucatán*, February 1911.

60. *La Revista Médica de Yucatán*, January 1924.

61. *La Revista Médica de Yucatán*, February 1940.

62. McCrea, *Diseased Relations*, 85, 109–13.

63. Martínez Cortés and Maretínez Barbosa, *El Consejo Superior de Salubridad*, 156.

64. *La Revista Médica de Yucatán*, February 1950.

65. For an official account of this process, see http://www.salud.yucatan.gob.mx/content/view/29/32/ (Accessed December 21, 2011).

66. Julyan G. Peard, *Race, Place, and Medicine: The Idea of the Tropics in Nineteenth-Century Brazilian Medicine* (Durham: Duke University Press, 1999); Julia Rodríguez, *Civilizing Argentina: Science, Medicine, and the Modern State* (Chapel Hill: The University of North Carolina Press, 2006).

67. Stepan, *Beginnings of Brazilian Science*.

Glossary

Ah-menes (h-men, singular)—Maya healers and spiritual leaders

Aljibe—below ground cistern in which many municipal residents stored water

Ayuntamiento—Spanish municipal organization; akin to a city council

Botica/boticario—pharmacy, could be independent, or associated with a hospital

Cah—Maya community of the pre-Columbian and colonial eras

Casta divina—the "divine caste" of the henequen era; group of some forty families with tremendous economic, social, and political power

Cenote—water-filled sinkhole, often associated with religious power in the pre-Columbian and colonial eras

Charlatan—a term used by biomedical physicians to label a healer who claimed more knowledge that he or she actually had; often claimed a scientific background

Curanderos—lay healer who often reflected a mix of indigenous and Hispanic methods

DSP—the Federal Department of Public Health, founded in 1917

Dzules—Maya term for foreigners, usually applied to whites

Ejidos—collectively held lands, originally given to indigenous communities by Spaniards; in the 1930s a major dimension of revolutionary agrarian reform

Henequeneros de Yucatán—1938–1955; an association of ejido members, henequen production and sales; and agrarian development. Power resided with former estate owners; its social assistance division developed an extensive public health system

Hospital O'Horan—Mérida's main hospital, modernized in 1906

Jefes políticos—political bosses; usually the head of a municipal government

Junta Superior de Sanidad—General Board of Health formed in 1894; Backbone of Yucatán's public health system.

Médicos—university-trained physicians, usually practiced biomedicine

Milpa—a "slash and burn" pattern of agriculture that is used for two or three years, and then rotated to a more fertile plot

Protomedicato—colonial medical licensing board that regulates titlted physicians and pharmacists

Puuc region—hill region that transverses center of Yucatán. Its thicker soils allow for a greater range of agricultural products, including corn and fruits

SSA—Secretaría de Salubridad y Asistencia. Formed by the Mexican government in 1943

Tienda—small neighborhood shop that often sells aspirins and other biomedical drugs

Vocales—medical officials that represent segments of a city, akin to "ward" physicians

Bibliography

ARCHIVES

Archivo General del Estado de Yucatán, Mérida, Mexico
Fondo Poder Ejecutivo
Sección Beneficencia
Serie Correspondencia
Serie Junta Superior de Sanidad
Serie Salubridad
Serie Sanidad
Sección Beneficencia y Sanidad
Serie Junta Superior de Sanidad
Sección Gobernación
Serie Correspondencia
Sección Junta Superior de Sanidad
Serie Copiador de Oficios
Archivo General de la Nación, Mexico City
Fondo Banco Nacional de Crédito S. A. (Yucatán)
Fondo Secretaría de Salubridad y Asistencia
Sección Departamento de Salubridad Pública
Sección Comisión Constructora
Sección Epidemiologia
Sección Dirección General de Servicios Coordinados de Salud Pública en Estados y Territorios
Presidential wings
Archivo Histórico de la Escuela de Medicina, Mexico City
Archivo Histórico de la Secretaría de Salubridad y Asistencia, Mexico City
Fondo Salubridad Pública
Sección Congresos y Convenciones
Sección Ejercicio de la Medicina

Sección Epidemiología
Sección Jurídica
Sección Presidencia
Sección Salubridad en Territorios, Puertos y Fronteras
Sección Secretaría
Fondo Secretaría de Salubridad y Asistencia
Sección Subsecretaría de Salubridad y Asistencia
Biblioteca del Museo de Antropología e Historia, Mexico City
Casa de Historia de Educación de Yucatán, Archivo Histórico
College of Physicians of Philadelphia, Historical Medical Library, Philadelphia, Pennsylvania
Biblioteca Yucatense, La Hemeroteca del Estado "José María Pino Suárez," Mérida, Mexico Library of Congress, Washington, DC
Philip S. Hench Walter Reed Yellow Fever On-line Collection, Historical Collections and Services, The Claude Moore Health Sciences Library, University of Virginia.
Rockefeller Foundation Archives, Rockefeller Archive Center, Sleepy Hollow, New York
National Archives and Records Administration, College Park, Maryland
Record Group 90 Records of the Public Health Service
General Subject File, 1924–1935
Foreign Governments, Mexico
National Library of Medicine, Bethesda, Maryland

NEWSPAPERS

Boletín Estadística, Mérida
Boletín de Higiene, Mérida
Boletín Mensual del Sindicato de Médicos y Profesionistas Conexos de Yucatán, Mérida
La Crónica Médica de Yucatán, Mérida
La Emulación, Mérida
La Higiene, Mérida
La Revista Médica de Yucatán, Mérida
Revista de Medicina Homeopática, Mérida

OTHER PRIMARY MATERIALS

"Acta de la Sesión Celebrada por la Comisión Especial para la Campaña contra la Fiebre Amarilla, Octubre 19 de 1921, Presidencia del Sr. Dr. T. C. Lyster." In *Memorias de la Primera Convención de Fiebre Amarilla, Octubre 15–20 de 1921*, 155–63. México DF: Departamento de Salubridad Pública, 1921.
Baz, Gustavo. *Secretaría de Salubridad y Asistencia, Memoria, 1943–44*. México DF: Estados Unidos Mexicanos, 1944.

Código sanitario del Estado de Yucatán. Mérida: Imprenta de la "Escuela Correccional de Artes y Oficios," 1911.

Congreso Médico Peninsular. *Segundo Congreso Médico Peninsular*. Mérida: Diaz Massa, 1945.

¿Cuales deben ser las medidas más adecuadas para prosequir la campaña contra el charlatanismo en sus diversas formas? Mérida: Sociedad Médica Yucateca, 1931.

Departamento de Salubridad Pública. *Informe general del Departamento de Salubridad que comprende las labores a cabo durante la administración de C. Lic. Emilio Portes Gil, siendo Jefe del Departamento el C. Dr. Aquilino Villanueva*. Mexico: Talleres del Imp. del Departamento de Salubridad Pública, 1930.

Departamento de Salubridad Pública. *Los servicios de higiene rural y medicina social*. México DF: Artes Gráficos del Estado, S. C. I., 1941.

Departamento de Salubridad Pública. *Memoria annual del Departamento de Salubridad Pública correspondiente al periodo Septiembre 1 de 1942–Agosto 31 de 1943*. México DF: Talleres Tipográficos Modelo, S. A., 1943.

Departamento de Salubridad Pública. *Memoria del Departamento de Salubridad Pública de Servicios Sanitarios Coordinados en los estados y territorias*. México DF: Artes Gráficas del Estado, S.C.L., 1940/1941.

Departamento de Salubridad Pública. *La Oficina Central de Higiene Rural y Servicios Coordinados en los estados*. México DF: Talleres del Imp. del Departamento de Salubridad Pública, 1937.

Departamento de Salubridad Pública. *Rural Hygiene and Social Medicine Services of the Department of Public Health: Organization-Functions, Results Obtained until 1940*. México DF: DSP, 1941.

Departamento de la Secretaría de Salubridad y Asistencia Pública. *Memoria de la Secretaría de Salubridad y Asistencia Pública. Sexencio* 1952–1958. México DF: Impreso por ACMEX, S. A., 1958.

El Hospital del Niño. Mérida: Gobierno del Estado de Yucatán, 1940.

Expedición de la Escuela de Medicina Tropical de Liverpool, 1911–1912. *Informe de la expedición para investigar la fiebre amarilla en Yucatán, por el Dr. HARALD SEIDELIN*. Mérida: Imprenta "el Porvenir," 1914.

Henequeneros de Yucatán. Departamento de Asistencia Social. *Asistencia Social*. Mérida. (serial publication, 1948–1951).

Henequeneros de Yucatán. *Documentos correspondientes a la Asamblea General Ordinaria de la Asociación denominada Henequeneros de Yucatán*. Mérida: Talleres Gráficas del Sudeste, S. A., 1939.

Henequeneros de Yucatán. *Informe general del comité directivo de la sociedad cooperativa de responsabilidad limitada "Henequeneros de Yucatán."* Mérida: Talleres de la Cia. Tipográfica Yucateca, S. A., 1928.

Henequeneros de Yucatán. *Informe del Consejo Directivo de Henequeneros de Yucatán, correspondiente del ejercicito de 1950*. Mérida: Editorial "Zamna," 1950.

Informe del Ciudadano Profesor José Gutiérrez Beytia, Gobernador Constitucional del Estado, año de 1948. Mérida: Gobierno del Estado de Yucatán, 1949.

Informe del Ciudadano Profesor José Gutiérrez Beytia, Gobernador Constitucional del Estado, año de 1949. Mérida: Talleres Gráficos, Edit. Zamorá, 1949.

Informe de Señor Ernesto Novelo Torres, Gobernador constitucional de Yucatán ante la XXXVI Legislatura del Estado, 1944. Mérida: Imprenta del Estado, 1945.

Informe rendido al gobernador constitucional de Yucatán c. Dr. Alvaro Torre Díaz, ante la XXIX Legislatura del Estado el 1° de Enero de 1927. Mérida: Talleres Tipográficos del Gobierno del Estado, 1927.

Informe rendido al gobernador constitucional de Yucatán c. Dr. Alvaro Torre Díaz, ante la XXX Legislatura del Estado el 1° de Enero de 1928. Mérida: Talleres Tipográficos del Gobierno del Estado, 1928.

Informe del Sr. Ingeniero Humberto Canto E., Gobernador Constitucional de Yucatán ante la XXIV legislatura del estado 1939. Mérida: Imprenta del Estado, 1940.

Memoria de la Secretaría de Salubridad y Asistencia Pública. Sexenio 1952–1958. México DF: Impreso for ACMEX, S. A., 1958.

Memoria, 1946–1951*, Departamento de Asistencia Social de Henequeneros de Yucatán*. Mérida: Henequeneros de Yucatán, 1952.

Oficina Central de Higiene Rural y Servicios Sanitarios en el Departamento de Salubridad Pública. *Directorio general*. México DF: NP, 1937.

Reglamento del Hospital General de esta capital. Mérida: Imprenta de Manuel Aldana Rivas, 1869.

Reglamento de la Sociedad Médico-Homeopática de Yucatán. Mérida: Imprenta "El Porvenir," 1922.

Reglamento para el gobierno interior del Hospital General San Juan de Dios de esta capital. Mérida: Imprenta Literaria a cargo de M. Guzmán, 1869.

Secretaría de Salubridad y Asistencia. Dirección General de los Servicios Médicos Rurales Cooperativos. *Organización y funcionamiento de los Servicios Médicos Rurales Cooperativos*. México DF: SSA, 1951.

Siurob, José. *Memoria del Departamento de Salubridad Pública de Septiembre de 1935 a Agosto de 1936*. México DF: D. A. P. P., 1937.

ARTICLES, BOOKS, AND DISSERTATIONS

Adams, Walter Randolph, and John P. Hawkins. *Health Care in Guatemala: Confronting Medical Pluralism in a Developing Country*. Norman: University of Oklahoma Press, 2007.

Agostoni, Claudia. "Médicos científicos y médicos ilícitos en la ciudad de México durante el Porfiriato." In *Estudios de Historia Moderna y Contemporánea de México* 19 (2000): 13–31. México DF: Universidad Nacional Autónoma de México, 1999.

———. *Monuments of Progress: Modernization and Public Health in Mexico City,* 1876–1910. Calgary: University of Calgary Press, 2003.

Aguilar Gómez, Eduardo. "El problema de la lucha anti-tuberculosa en Yucatán: Base para abordarlo." In Congreso Médico Peninsular. *Memorias del segundo congreso médico peninsular*, 280–87. Mérida: Díaz Massa, 1945.

Aguilar Sarmiento, Samuel. *La asistencia social en el ejido henequenero de Yucatán*. Mérida: NP, 1953.

Aguirre Beltrán, Gonzalo. *Medicina y magia. El proceso de aculturación en la estructura colonial.* México DF: Instituto Indigenista, 1963.

———. Gonzalo. *Programas de salud en la situación intercultural.* México DF: INI, 1955.

Alvárez Amezquita, José, Miguel E. Bustamante, Antonio López Picazos, and Francisco Fernández del Castillo. *Historia de la Salubridad y de la Asistencia en México.* 4 vols. México DF: Secretaría de Salubridad y Asistencia, 1960.

Antochiw, Michel. *Los santos y las enfermedades de nuestros abuelos.* Mérida: Compañía Editorial de la Península, S. A. de C. V, 2001.

Anzures y Bolaños, María del Carmen. *La Medicina Tradicional en México: Proceso Histórico Sincretismos, y Conflictos.* México DF: UNAM, 1983.

Arzápalo Marín, Ramón. *El Ritual de los bacabes: edición facsimilar, Fuentes para el Estudio de la cultura Maya 5.* México DF: Instituto de Investigaciones Filológicas, Centro de Estudios Mayas, Universidad Nacional Autónoma de México, 1987.

Armus, Diego, ed. *Disease in the History of Modern Latin America: From Malaria to AIDS.* Durham: Duke University Press, 2003.

———. "Disease in the Historiography of Modern Latin America." In *Disease in the History of Modern Latin America: From Malaria to AIDS*, ed. by Diego Armus, 1–24. Durham: Duke University Press, 2003.

———. *The Ailing City: Health, Tuberculosis, and Culture in Buenos Aires, 1870–1950.* Durham: Duke University Press, 2011.

Arnold, David. *Imperial Medicine and Indigenous Societies.* Manchester, UK: Manchester University Press, 1988.

Askinasy, Siegfried. *El problema agrario de Yucatan.* 2nd ed. México DF: Ediciones Botas, 1936.

Ayora-Díaz, Steffan Igor. "Globalization, Rationality and Medicine: Local Medicine's Struggle for Recognition in the Highland Chiapas, Mexico." *Urban Anthropology* 27:2 (1998): 165–95.

Ayuso y O'Horibe, Horcano. *Museo "Seidelin" (de Anatomía Patológica).* Mérida: Editorial del Gobierno del Estado de Yucatán, 1944.

Balam Pereira, Gilberto. *Cosmogonía y uso actual de las plantas medicinales de Yucatán.* Mérida: Ediciones de la Universidad Autónoma de Yucatán, 1992.

Baños Ramírez, Othón. *Campesinos y sociedad: Ayer y hoy.* Mérida: Ediciones de la Universidad Autónoma de Yucatán, 1996.

———. Othón. *La modernidad rural mexicana a fines de milenio. El caso de Yucatán.* Mérida: Universidad Autónoma de Yucatán, 2001.

Barry, John M. *The Great Influenza: The Epic Story of the Deadliest Plague in History.* New York: Penguin Books, 2004.

Benchimol, Jaime L., ed. *Manguihos, do sonho à vida: A ciência na Belle Époque.* Rio de Janeiro: Casa de Oswaldo Cruz, 1990.

Bendiner, Elmer. "Noguchi: Many Triumphs and a Brilliant Failure." *Hospital Practice* 19:2 (February 1984): 222–55.

Benevides García, Raymundo. *Historia de la salud pública de Nuevo León [1820–1950].* Monterrey: Universidad Autónoma de Nuevo León, 1998.

Betancourt Agramonte, Rafael. *Remitente Biliosa forma hemorrágica de a corre en los nativos de Yucatán.* Mérida: Tip. y Lit. "La Moderna," 1913.

Birn, Anne-Emanuelle. "A Revolution in Rural Health?: The Struggle over Local Health Units in Mexico, 1928–1940." *Journal of the History of Medicine and Allied Sciences* 53:1 (1998): 43–76.

———. "Healers, Healing, and Child Well-Being: Ideologies, Institutions, and Health in Latin America and the Caribbean." *Latin American Research Review* 40:2 (June 2005): 176–92.

———. *Marriage of Convenience: Rockefeller International Health and Revolutionary Mexico.* Rochester: University of Rochester Press, 2006.

———. "Revolution, the Scatological Way: The Rockefeller Foundation's Hookworm Campaign in 1920s Mexico." In *Disease in the History of Modern Latin America: From Malaria to AIDS*, Ed. by Diego Armus, 158–82. Durham: Duke University Press, 2003.

———. "Wa(i)ves of Influence: Rockefeller Public Health in Mexico, 1920–1950." *Studies in History and Philosophy of Biological and Biomedical Sciences* 31:3 (2000): 381–95.

——— and Raúl Neochochea López. "Footprints on the Future: Looking Forward to the History of Health and Medicine in the Twenty-First Century." *Hispanic American Historical Review* 91:3 (August 2011): 502–27.

Bliss, Katherine Elaine. *Compromised Positions: Prostitution, Public Health, and Gender Politics in Revolutionary Mexico City.* University Park: Pennsylvania State University Press, 2001.

Bloom, Khaled J. *The Mississippi Valley's Great Yellow Fever Epidemic of 1878.* Baton Rouge: Louisiana State University Press, 1993.

Bracamonte y Sosa, Pedro, and Gabriela Solís Robleda. *Espacios Mayas de autónomia: el pacto colonial en Yucatán.* Mérida: Universidad Autónoma de Yucatán, 1996.

Brachet de Márquez, Viviane. *The Dynamics of Domination: State, Class, and Social Reform in Mexico,* 1910–1990. Pittsburgh: University of Pittsburgh Press, 1994.

Brannon, Jeffery and Eric N. Baklanoff. *Agrarian Reform and Public Enterprise in Mexico: The Political Economy of Yucatán's Henequen Industry.* Tuscaloosa: The University of Alabama Press, 1987.

Brea, Jorge. "Population Dynamics in Latin America." *Population Bulletin*
58:1 (March 2003): 3–33.

Brown, Denise F. "Life in the Fast Lane: Change over three Generations in a Yucatec Maya Town." In *Maya Survivalism. Acta Mesoamericana* Vol. 12, 217–23. Verlag: Anton Saurwein, 2001.

Brown, Theodore M, Marcos Cueto, and Elixabeth Fee. "The World Health Organization and the Transition From 'International' to 'Global' Public Health." *American Journal of Public Health* 96:1 (2006): 62–72.

Brunhouse, Robert L. *Sylvanus G. Morley and the World of the Ancient Mayas.* Norman: University of Oklahoma Press, 1971.

Bustamante, Miguel E. *Cinco personajes de la salud en México.* México DF: Grupo Editorial Angel Porrúa, 1986.

———. "La Coordinación de los Servicios Sanitarios Federales y Locales Como Factor de Progreso Higiénico en México." *Gaceta Médica de México* 65 (1934): 179–228.

———. "La Coordinación de los Servicios Sanitarios Federales y Locales Como Factor de Progreso Higiénico en México." In *La Atención Médica en el Medio Rural Mexicano*. Edited by Héctor Hernández Llamas, 35–90. México, DF: IMSS, 1984.

———. "La coordinación de los Servicios sanitarios federales y locales como factor de progreso higiénico en México, su evolución y desarrollo de 1934 a 1964." In *Academia Nacional de Medicina. Libro Conmemorativo del Primer Centenario*. Tomo II, 652–64. México, DF: Academia Nacional de Medicina, 1964.

———. *La fiebre amarilla en México y su origen en America*. México DF: Instituto de Salubridad y Enfermedades Tropicales de la Secretaría de Salubridad y Asistencia, 1958.

———. "Public Health Administration in Latin America." *American Journal of Public Health* 40:9 (September 1950): 1067–71.

Cámara-Milán, Pedro. "El Dr. Hideyo Noguchi en Yucatán." *Revista Biomédica* 11 (2000): 207–212.

Campos García, Melchor. *De provincia a estado de la república Mexicana: La península de Yucatán, 1786–1835*. Mérida: Universidad Autónoma de Yucatán, Consejo Nacional de Ciencia y Tecnología, 2004.

Cárdenas, Lázaro. *Lázaro Cárdenas en Yucatán (1934–1937): Discursos*. Mérida: Gobierno del Estado de Yucatán, 1987.

Cárdenas, Rosario. "Las causas de muerte en México." In *La población de México: Tendencias y perspectivas sociodemográficas hacia el siglo XXI*. Coordinated by José Gómez de León Cruces and Cecilia Rabell Romero, 109–67. México DF: Consejo Nacional de Población, Fondo de Cultura Económica, 2001.

Carrillo Gil, Alvar. *Dos enfermedades por carencia en Yucatán*. Mérida. NP, 1935.

Carrillo, Ana María. "Los comienzos de la bacteriología en México." *Elementos: Ciencia y Cultura* 42:8 (June-August 2001), accessed September 16, 2003 at http://wwww.elementos.buap.mx/num42/htm/23.htm

———. "Los difíciles caminos de la campaña antivariolosa en México." *Ciencias* 55–56 (July to December, 1999): 18–25.

———. "Guerra de exterminio al 'Fantasma de las costas': La primera campaña contra la fiebre amarilla en México, 1903–1911." In *Curar, Sanar y Educar: Enfermedad y Sociedad en México Siglos XIX y XX*. Coordinated by Claudia Agostoni, 221–256. México DF: Universidad Nacional Autónoma de México; Benemérita Universidad Autónoma de Puebla, 2008.

———. "Economía, política y salud pública en el México porfiriano (1876–1910)." *História, Ciência, Saúde—Manguinhos* 9 (2002): 67–87.

———. "Médicos del México Decimonónico: Entre el Control Estatal y la Autonomía Profesional." *Dynamis* 22 (2002): 351–75.

———. "Nacimiento y Muerte de una Profesión: Las Parteras Tituladas en México." *Dynamis* 19 (1999): 167–90

Carroll, Patrick. *Science, Culture, and Modern State Formation.* Berkeley, CA: University of California Press, 2006.

Carter, Henry Rose. *Yellow Fever: An Epidemiological and Historical Study of its Place of Origin.* Baltimore: The Williams & Wilkins Company, 1931.

Case, Henry R. *Views on and of Yucatán Besides Notes upon parts of the state of Campeche and the Territory of Quintana Roo.* Mérida: Henry A. Case, 1911.

Caselli, Graziella France Meslé, and Jacques Vallin. "Epidemiologic Transition Theory Exceptions." *Genus* 58:1 (January-March 2002): 9–51.

Castillo Canché, Jorge I., and José E. Serrano Catzín. "Vigilar y normar el burdel: Legalización de la prostitución femenina en Yucatán durante el porfiriato." *Revista de la Universidad Autónoma de Yucatán* 198 (January, February, March 1994): 46–55.

Cevera-Andrade, Alejandro. "Harald Seidelin. Su labor in Yucatán, México." *Revista Biomédica* 17:3 (July–September 2002): 221–24.

________. "Apuntes para la historia del Hospital O'Horán de la ciudad de Mérida, Yucatán, México," *Revista Biomédica*, 12:1 (January–March 2001): 63–74. (Originally Published in the *Revista de la Universidad de Yucatán* Vol. 36 (1964): 11–29.)

Cervera Fernández, José Juan. "Preceptos divinos y contradicciones racionales: el primer movimiento espiritista en Yucatán, 1869–1879." In *Los Aguafiestas: Desafíos a la hegemonía de la élite yucateca, 1867–1910.* Coordinated by Piedad Peniche Rivero and Felipe Escalante Tió, 193–238. Mérida: AGEY, 2002.

Clark, Paul Franklin. "Hideyo Noguchi, 1876–1928." *Bulletin of the History of Medicine* 33:1 (January–February 1959): 1–20.

Clendinnen, Inga. *Ambivalent Conquests: Maya and Spaniard in Yucatán, 1517–1570,* 2nd ed. New York: Cambridge University Press, 2003.

Colomé T. Rafael. *La Escuela de Medicina Homeopática de Yucatán; Fundación, Actuación, y clausura.* Mérida: Talleres "Impresora Popular," 1938.

Congreso Médico Peninsular. *Memorias del segundo congreso médico peninsular.* Mérida: Díaz Massa, 1945.

Connor, M. E. "Acta de la Primera Sesión Plena, Octubre 15 de 1921." In *Memoria de la Primera Convención de Fiebre Amarilla, Octubre 15–20 de 1921.* México DF: DSP, 1921.

———. "Informe Preliminar Sobre la Campaña Contra la Fiebre Amarilla, en Mérida, Yuc." In *Memoria de la Primera Convención de Fiebre Amarilla, Octubre* 1–21 *de 1921*, 21–25. México DF: DSP, 1921.

Cook, Noble David. *Born to Die: Disease and New World Conquest, 1492–1650.* Cambridge: Cambridge University Press, 1998.

Cook, Sherburne F. and Woodrow Wilson Borah. "The Population of Yucatan." In *Essays in Population History: Mexico and the Caribbean*, Volume 2: 1–179. Berkeley: University of California Press, 1974.

Corner, George W. *A History of the Rockefeller Institute,* 1901–1953*: Origins and Growth.* New York: The Rockefeller Institute Press, 1964.

Crandon-Malamud, Libbet. *From the Fat of Our Souls: Social Change, Political Processes, and Medical Pluralism in Bolivia.* Berkeley: University of California Press, 1991.

Crosby Jr., Alfred W. *The Columbian Exchange: Biological and Cultural Consequences of 1492*. Westport, CT: Greenwood Press, 1972.

Crosby, Molly Caldwell. *The American Plague: The Untold Story of Yellow Fever. The Epidemic that Shaped our History*. New York: Berkley Books, 2006.

Cruz, Martín de la. *The de la Cruz-Badiano Aztec Herbal of 1552*. Trans. by William Gates. Baltimore: The Maya Society, 1939.

Cuenya Mateo, Miguel Ángel. *Puebla de los Ángeles en tiempos de una peste colonial. Una mirada en torno al matlazahuatl de 1737*. Puebla: Benemérita Universidad Autónoma de Puebla and El Colegio de Michoacán, 1999.

Cuenya Mateo, Miguel Ángel, coordinator. *Cabildo, sociedad y política sanitaria en la ciudad de Puebla, 1750–1910*. Puebla: Benemérita Universidad Autónoma de Puebla, 2003.

Cueto, Marcos. *Cold War, Deadly Fevers: Malaria Eradication in Mexico, 1955–1975*. Washington, DC: Woodrow Wilson Center Press, The Johns Hopkins University Press, 2007.

———. "The cycles of eradication: The Rockefeller Foundation and Latin American Public Health." In *International health organisations and movements, 1918–1939*. Ed. by Paul Weindling, 222–43. Cambridge: Cambridge University Press, 1995.

———. *The Value of Heath: A History of the Pan American Health Organization*. Washington, DC: Pan American Health Organization, 2007.

Cueto, Marcos, ed. *Missionaries of Science: The Rockefeller Foundation and Latin America*. Bloomington: Indiana University Press, 1994.

Cueto, Marcos, and Steven Palmer. *Medicine and Public Health in Latin America: A History*. New York: Cambridge University Press, 2014.

De Landa, Diego. *Yucatán Before and After the Conquest*. Trans. By William Gates, 2nd ed. Baltimore: The Maya Society, 1937.

Delaporte, François, *The History of Yellow Fever: An Essay on the Birth of Tropical Medicine*. Trans. by Arthur Goldhammer. Cambridge: The MIT Press, 1991.

Díaz, José F., and Benjamín Gongora Triay. "La higiene." In *Enciclopedia Yucatanese*. Tomo VI, 377–421. 2nd ed. Mérida: Edición Oficial del Gobierno de Yucatán, 1977.

Dr. Eduardo Urzaiz Rodríguez. Mérida: Ediciones de la Universidad de Yucatán.

Dubin, Martin David. "The League of Nations Health Organisation." In *International Health, Organisations, and Movements, 1918–1939*. Ed. by Paul Weindling, 56–80. Cambridge: Cambridge University Press, 1995.

Duffy, John. *The Sanitarians: A History of American Public Health*. Chicago: University of Illinois Press, 1990.

Dumond, Don E. *The Machete and the Cross: Campesino Rebellion in Yucatán*. Lincoln: University of Nebraska Press, 1997.

Durán Córdova, José. *Organización y funcionamiento de los Servicios Médicos Cooperativos Ejidales*. México DF, 1951. (Mimeograph prepared for a meeting of the Asociación Fronteriza México-Norteamericano de Salubridad Pública, Los Angeles, CA).

Echeverría V., Pedro. *La política en Yucatán en el siglo XX, 1900–1964*. Mérida: Maldonado Editores, 1985.

Edmonson, Munro S. and Victoria R. Bricker. "Yucatecan Mayan Literature." In *Supplement to the Handbook of Middle American Indians. Volume Three. Literatures*. Ed. by Munro S. Edmonson, 44–63. Austin: University of Texas Press, 1985.

Eiss, Paul. *In the Name of the Pueblo: Place, Community, and the Politics of History in Yucatán*. Durham: Duke University Press, 2010.

Erosa Barbachano, Arturo. *Biografía del Dr. Agustín Jorge O'Horan Escudero*. Mérida: Ediciones de la Universidad Autónoma de Yucatán, 2005.

———. *La Escuela de Medicina de Mérida, Yucatán*. Mérida: Ediciones de la Universidad Autónoma de Yucatán, 1997.

———. "Necesidad de pequeños hospitales rurales." In *Memorias del segundo congreso médico peninsular* , 266–67. Mérida: Díaz Massa, 1945.

———. *Vida y obra del Doctor Vado*. Mérida: Ediciones de la Universidad Autónoma de Yucatán, 1995.

Erosa Cámara, Mario. *Epistolario de un médico*. Mérida: Maldonado Editores, 1984.

Espinosa, Mariola. *Epidemic Invasions: Yellow Fever and the Limits of Cuban Independence, 1878–1930*. Chicago: The University of Chicago Press, 2009.

Fallaw, Ben. *Cárdenas Compromised: The Failure of Reform in Postrevolutionary Yucatán*. Durham, NC: Duke University Press, 2001.

———. 'The Germ of Fanaticism: Science and Anticlericalism in Postrevolutionary State Formation in Mexico, c. 1915–1940." Paper presented to the LASA International Congress, Toronto, Canada, October 7th, 2010.

Farfán López, Emiliano. "Problemas asistenciales de los Ejidatarios de Yucatán." *Clínica Médico Quirúrgica* 6 (1944): 144–53.

Farriss, Nancy M. *Maya Society under Colonial Rule: the Collective Enterprise of Survival*. Princeton: Princeton University Press, 1984.

Fenner, Frank et al. *Smallpox and Its Eradication*. Geneva: World Health Organization, 1988.

Few, Roger, Alfonso Mercado, Boris Graizbord, Lilian Albornoz Mendoz. *Climatic Hazards, Health Risk and Response, Case Study 4: Yucatán, Mexico*. London: UK Economic and Research Council, January 2008.

Fidler, David. "The Globalization of Public Health: The First 100 Years of International Health Diplomacy." *Bulletin of the World Health Organization* 79 (2000): 842–49.

Finkler, Kaja. "Sacred Healing and Biomedicine Compared." *Medical Anthropology Quarterly* 8:2 (1994): 178–97.

Finlay, Carlos E. *Carlos Finlay and Yellow Fever*. New York: The Institute of Tropical Medicine of the University of Havana, Oxford University Press, 1940.

Fisher, Donald. "Rockefeller Philanthropy and the British Empire: The Creation of the London School of Hygiene and Tropical Medicine." *History of Education* 7 (1978): 129–43.

Foucault, Michael. *The Birth of the Clinic: An Archeology of Medical Perception*. Trans. A. M. Sheridan Smith. New York: Vintage/Random House, 1994.

———. *The History of Sexuality: The Will to Knowledge,* Volume 1. New York: Random House, 1990.

Fuentes Gómez, José Humberto, and Magnolia Rosado Lugo. "Mérida: La obra urbana en el porfiriato." In *Identidades sociales en Yucatán*. Compiled by María Cecilia Lara Cebada, 71–98. Mérida: Universidad Autónoma de Yucatán, Facultad de Ciencias Antropológicas, 1997.

Gamio, Manuel. *Algunos consideraciones sobre la salubridad y la demografía en México. Contribución de la Secretaria de Gobernación a la Conferencia Inter-Americana de Higiene Rural*. México DF: DAPP, 1939.

Gillespie, James A. "Europe, America, and the Space of International Health." In *Shifting Boundaries of Public Health: Europe in the Twentieth Century*. Ed. by Susan Gross Soloman, Lion Murard, and Patrick Zylberman, 114–137. Rochester: University of Rochester Press, 2008.

Gobierno del Estado de Yucatán. *El ejido henequenero de Yucatán. Su historia desde el 1° de Febrero de 1938 hasta el 30 de Noviembre de 1940*. Segunda Parte. Mérida: Editorial Cultura, 1941.

Golden, Grace. "Juan de Dios and the Hospital of Christian Charity." *Journal of the History of Medicine and Allied Sciences* 33:1 (1978): 6–34.

Goldstein, Michael, and Peter Donaldson. "Exporting Professionalism: A Case Study of Medical Education." *Journal of Health and Social Behavior* 20 (1979): 322–37.

Gómez-Dantés, Octavio. "Health Reform and Policies for the Poor in Mexico." In *Health Reform and Poverty in Latin America*. Ed. P. Lloyd-Sherlock, 128–142. London: Institute of Latin American Studies, University of London, 2000.

Gonzáles, Michael J. *The Mexican Revolution, 1910–1940*. Albuquerque: University of New Mexico Press, 2002.

González Beytia, José. "La asistencia social y la salubridad en Yucatán, durante 1948." *Asistencia Social* 3 (January-February-March 1949), 42–49.

González Leandri, Ricard. "La profesión médica en Buenos Aires, 1852–1870." In *Política, médica y enfermedades. Lecturas de historia de la salud en la Argentina*. Ed. by Mirta Zaida Lobato, 21–53. Buenos Aires: Editorial Biblos, 1996.

González Navarro, Moisés. *Raza y tierra: La guerra de castas y el henequén*. México DF: El Colegio de México, 1970.

Goodman, Margaret. "Does Political Corruption Really Help Economic Development?: Yucatán, Mexico." *Polity* 7:2 (Winter 1974): 143–63.

Grant, Martha. "Influencia de las Costumbres y Creencias Populares en los Servicios de un Centro de Salud." *Boletín de la Oficina Sanitaria Panamericana* 33 (1952): 283–97.

Graves, Charles. *Invasion by Virus: Can it Happen Again*? London: Icon Books Limited, 1969.

Grupo Dzíbil. Sociedad Mexicana de Geografía y Estadística. *El libro de los médicos yerbateros de Yucatán*. Mérida: Compañía Editorial Impresora y Distribuidora, S. A., 1997.

Gruzinski, Serge. *The Mestizo Mind: The Intellectual Dynamics of Colonization and Globalization*. Trans. by Deke Dusinberre. New York: Routledge, 2002.

Gubler, Ruth. "La medicina tradicional en Yucatán a través de los siglos." In *Yucatán a través de los siglos* (Memorias del 49th Congreso Internacional de Americanistas,

Quito, Ecuador, 1997). Organized by Ruth Gubler, 229–47. Mérida: Universidad Autónoma de Yucatán, 2001.

Güémez Pineda, Miguel A. "De comadronas a promotoras de salud y planificación familiar: Proceso de incorporación de las parteras empíricas Yucatecas al sistema institucional de salud." In *Cambio cultural y resocialización en Yucatán*. Coordinated by Estebán Krotz, 117–45. Mérida: Ediciones de la Universidad Autónoma de Yucatán, 1997.

Guerra, Francisco. "Maya Medicine." *Medical History* 8:1 (January 1964): 31–43.

———. "Pre-Columbian Medicine: Its Influence on Medicine Today." In *Aspects of the History of Medicine in Latin America*. Ed. by John Z. Bowers and Elizabeth F. Purcell, 1–15. New York: Josiah Macy Jr. Foundation, 1979.

Gurri, Francisco D., Gilberto Balam Pereira, Emilio F. Moran. "Well-Being Changes in Response to 30 Years of Regional Integration in Maya Populations from Yucatán, Mexico." *American Journal of Human Biology* 15 (2001): 590–602.

Gutiérrez Rivas, Efraím. *Dr. Harald Seidelin. Su obra en Yucatán y algunas de sus actividades en otros lugares*. Mérida: Diaz Massa, 1951.

Guy, Donna J. "Medical Imperialism Gone Awry: The Campaign Against Legalized Prostitution in Latin America." In Meade and Walker, eds. *Science, Medicine and Cultural Imperialism*, 75–94. New York: St. Martin's Press, 1991.

Guzmán Medina, María Guadelupe Violeta. "Dinámica social, salud y poder: Un análisis antropológico de las concepciones ideológicas de la salud y enfermedad en una comunidad Maya de Yucatán." In *Identidades sociales en Yucatán*. Compiled by María Cecilia Lara Cebada, 135–157. Mérida: Universidad Autónoma de Yucatán, Facultad de Ciencias Antropológicas, 1997.

Hamilton, Nora. *The Limits of State Autonomy: Post-Revolutionary Mexico*. Princeton, NJ: Princeton University Press, 1982.

Hansen, Asael T. "Change in the Class System of Mérida, Yucatán, 1875–1935." In *Yucatán: A World Apart*. Ed. by Edward H. Mosely and Edward D. Terry, 122–41. University, AL: The University of Alabama Press, 1980.

________. "Mérida y el interior del estado." In *Enciclopedia Yucatanense*. Ed. by Francisco Luna Kan, Luis H. Hoyos Villanueva, and Carlos A. 2nd ed., 423–453. México: Gobierno de Yucatán, 1977.

Hansen, Asael T., and Juan R. Bastarrachea M. *Mérida: Su transformación: de capital colonial a naciente metrópolis*. México: Instituto Nacional de Antropología e Historia, 1984.

Harman, Robert Charles. *Cambios médicos y sociales en una comunidad maya-tzeltal*. México DF: Instituto Nacional Indigenista y Secretaría de Educación Pública, 1974.

Hartesveldt, Fred R. van, ed. *The 1918–1919 Pandemic of Influenza: The Urban Impact on the Western World*. Lewiston, NY: The Edwin Mellen Press, 1992.

Hays, J. N. *The Burdens of Disease: Epidemics and Human Response in Western History*. New Brunswick, NJ: Rutgers University Press, 1998.

Haynes, Douglas M. *Imperial Medicine: Patrick Manson and the Conquest of Tropical Disease*. Philadelphia: University of Pennsylvania Press, 2001.

Hernández Sáenz, Luz María. *Learning to Heal: The Medical Profession in Colonial Mexico*, 1767–1831. New York: Peter Lang, 1997.

Hernández, Luz María, and George M. Foster. "Curers and Their Cures in Colonial New Spain and Guatemala: The Spanish Component." In *Mesoamerican Healers*. Ed. by Brad R. Huber and Alan R. Sandstrom, 19–46. Austin: Texas University Press, 2001.

Hernández Llamas, Héctor. "La atención médica en el medio rural mexicano." In Hector Hernández Llamas, compiler, *La atención médica rural en México, 1930–1980*. México DF: Instituto Mexicano de Seguro Social, 1984.

Hernández Llamas, Héctor. "Historia de la Participación del Estado en las Instituciones de Atención Médica en México, 1935–1980." In *Vida y Muerte del Mexicano*. Edited by Federico Ortiz Quesada, 49–96. México DF: Folios Ediciones, 1982.

Hervik, Peter. *Mayan People Within and Beyond Boundaries: Social Categories and Lived Identity in Yucatán*. Amsterdam: Harwood Academic Publishers, 1999.

———. "The Mysterious Maya of National Geographic." *Journal of Latin American Anthropology* 4:1 (1999): 166–97.

Homedes, Núria, and Atonio Ugalde. *Decentralizing Health Services in Mexico: A Case Study in State Reform*. La Jolla, CA: Center for US – Mexican Studies, UCSD, 2006.

Honigsbaum, Mark. *The Fever Trail: In Search of the Cure for Malaria*. New York: Farrar, Straus and Giroux, 2001.

Horn, James. "The Mexican Revolution and Health Care or the Health of the Mexican Revolution." *International Journal of Health Services* 15:3 (1985): 485–99.

Hostettler, Ueli, and Matthew Restall, eds. *Maya Survivalism*. Acta MesoAmericana. Volume 12. Verlag: Anton Saurwein, 2001.

Iturbide Alvirex, Salvador. "Panorama General de la Salubridad Pública en México." *Pasteur: Revista Mensual de Medicina* 10, II, no. 4 (1973): 93–102.

Instituto Mexicano del Seguro Social. *Diagnóstico de salud en las zonas marginadas rurales de México*. México DF: Instituto Mexicano del Seguro Social, 1983.

Johnson, Niall P. A. S., and Juergen Mueller. "Updating the Accounts: Global Mortality of the 1918–1920 'Spanish' Influenza Pandemic." *Bulletin of the History of Medicine* 76:1 (Spring 2002): 105–15.

Jones, Grant D. *Maya Resistance to Spanish Rule: Time and History on a Colonial Frontier*. Albuquerque: University of New Mexico Press, 1989.

Joseph, Gilbert M. and Daniel Nugent, eds. *Everyday Forms of State Formation: Revolution and the Negotiation of Rule in Modern Mexico*. Durham: Duke University Press, 1994.

"Juan de Dios," *Diccionario de historia eclesiástica de España*, 4 vols. Madrid: NP, 1972), II, 1248–49.

Kapelusz-Poppi, Ana María. "Physician Activists and the Development of Rural Health in Postrevolutionary Mexico." *Radical History Review* 80 (Spring 2001): 35–50.

———. "Rural Health and State Construction in Post-Revolutionary Mexico: The Nicolaita Project for Rural Medical Services." *The Americas* 58:2 (October 2001): 261–83.

Kipple, Kenneth F., and Brian T. Higgins. "Yellow Fever and the Africanization of the Caribbean." In *Disease and Demography in the Americas*. Ed. by John W. Verano and Douglas H. Ubelaker, 238–41. Washington: Smithsonian Institution Press, 1992.

Knaut, Andrew Louis. "Disease and the Late Colonial Public Health Initiative in the Atlantic Ports of New Spain." (Ph. D. diss., Duke University, 1994).

Kocyba, Henryk Karol. "La Medicina y la Religión entre los Mayas Prehispánicos." In *Historia de la Salud en México,* 13–26. México DF: INAH, 1996.

Koivusalo, Meri, and Eeva Ollila. *Making a Healthy World: Agencies, Actors and Policies in International Health.* London: Zed Press, 1997.

Koss-Chioino, Joan D., Thomas Leatherman, and Christine Greenway eds. *Medical Pluralism in the Andes.* New York: Routledge, 2003.

Kunow, Mariana Appel. *Maya Medicine: Traditional Healing in Yucatán.* Albuquerque: University of New Mexico Press, 2003.

Lanning, John Tate. *The Royal Protomedicato: The Regulation of the Medical Professions in the Spanish Empire.* Ed. by John Jay TePaske. Durham: Duke University Press, 1985.

Larson, Brooke. *Trials of Nation Making: Liberalism, Race, and Ethnicity in the Andes, 1810–1910.* New York: Cambridge University Press, 2004.

Lasso Echerverría, Fernando. *Historia de los Servicios de salud en el Estado de Guerrero.* México DF: Impresores Especiales, 2003.

Lewis, Stephen E. "Mexico's National Indigenist Institute and the Negotiation of Applied Anthropology in Highland Chiapas, 1951–1954." *Ethnohistory* 55:4 (Fall 2008): 609–32.

López Aguilar, Verónica Marisol, Lía Esther Pérez Guerra, and Marco Antonio Sánchez Solís. *De la superstición a la ciencia: la enfermería universitaria en Yucatán.* Mérida: FEUADY, 2003.

López-Denis, Adrián. "Comments on the Panel "Between Foreign Approaches and Domestic Priorities: The Forging of International Health in Twentieth Century Latin America." (Presented at the XXIX International Congress of the Latin American Studies Association, Toronto Canada, October 6–9, 2010).

Löwy, Ilana. "Epidemiology, Immunology, and Yellow Fever: The Rockefeller Foundation in Brazil, 1923–1939." *Journal of the History of Biology* 30 (1997): 397–417.

Lozoya, Xavier, and Carlos Zolla, eds. *La Medicina Invisible: Introducción al Estudio de la Medicina Tradicional de México.* México DF: Folios Ediciones, 1983.

Luttrell, Anthony. "The Earliest Hospitallers." In *Montjoie: Studies in Crusade History in Honour of Hans Eberhard Mayer.* Ed. by Benjamin Z. Kedar, Jonathan Riley-Smith, and Rudolf Hiestand. Aldershot, 37–54. England: Ashgate Publishing, 1997.

Lutz, Catherine A., and Jane L. Collins. *Reading National Geographic.* Chicago: University of Chicago Press, 1993.

Madsen, Claudia. "A Study of Change in Mexican Folk Medicine." In *Contemporary Latin American Culture.* Ed. by Munro S. Edmonson, Claudia Madsen, and Jane Fishburne Collier, 89–137. New Orleans: Middle American Research Institute, Tulane University, 1968.

Malvado, Elsa, and Miguel Ángel Cuenya. "La Pandemia de Cólera de 1833 en la Ciudad de Puebla." In *El Cólera de 1833: Una Nueva Patología en México. Causas y Efectos.* Ed. by Miguel Ángel Cuenya et al., 11–45. México DF: INAH, 1992.

Malvado, Elsa, and Maria Elena Morales, eds. *Historia de la Salud en México.* México DF: INAH, 1996.

Marentes Miranda, Tomás. *Reseña histórica, geográfica y estadísticas del Estado de Yucatán.* México: SN, 1951.

Mark, Catherine, and José G. Rigau-Pérez. "The World's First Immunization Campaign: The Spanish Smallpox Vaccine Expedition, 1803–1813." *Bulletin of the History of Medicine* 83:1 (Spring 2009): 63–94.

Martínez Barbosa, Xóchitl, Fernando Martínez Cortés, Octavio Rivero Serrano. *Consejo de Salubridad General: la explicación histórica de su evolución y las reflexiones sobre su situación actual,* 1939–2000. México DF: SmithKline Beecham Mexico, Casa de Vacunas, 2000.

Martínez Cortés, Fernando. *La medicina científica y el siglo XIX mexicano.* México DF: Fondo de Cultura Económica, 1987.

Martínez Cortés, Fernando, and Xóchitl Martínez Barbosa. *El Consejo Superior de Salubridad. Rector de Salud Pública en México.* México DF: SmithKline Beecham Mexico, 1997.

Márquez, Patricio V., and Daniel J. Joly. "A Historical Overview of the Ministries of Public Health and the Medical Programs of the Social Security Systems in Latin America." *Journal of Public Health Policy* 7 (1986): 378–94.

Mazzaferri, Anthony. *Public Health and Social Revolution in Mexico:* 1870–1930. (Ph. D. diss., Kent State University, 1968).

McCrea, Heather. *Diseased relations: Epidemics, public health, and state formation in nineteenth-century Yucatan, Mexico.* (Ph. D. diss., State University of New York at Stony Brook, 2002).

———. Heath. *Diseased Relations: Epidemics, Public Health, and State-Building in Yucatán, Mexico,* 1847–1924. Albuquerque: University of New Mexico Press, 2011.

———. "White Man's Medicine: Smallpox Vaccination Campaigns in Mexico's Yucatán Peninsula."(Paper presented at the Latin American Studies Association, Miami Florida, March 2000).

McLeod, James Angus. "Public Health, Social Assistance and the Consolidation of the Mexican state: 1877–1940." (Ph. D. dissertation, Tulane University, 1990).

Memoria de la Primera Convención de Fiebre Amarilla, Octubre 15–20 *de 1921.* México DF: DSP, 1921

Méndez, Marciano Netzhualcoyotzil. "La Influenza de 1918 en Tlaxcala: Mortalidad y Efectos Sociales." *Boletín Mexicana de Historia y Filosofía de Medicina* 6:1 (2003): 23–31.

Mendiola Gómez, Jaime. "Historical Synthesis of Medical Education in Mexico." In *Aspects of the History of Medicine in Latin America.* Ed. by John Z. Powers and Elizabeth F. Purcell, 88–96. New York: Josiah Macy, Jr. Foundation, 1979.

Menéndez, Eduardo L. *Antropología médica. Orientaciones, desigualidades, y tranacciones.* México DF: Cuadernos de la Casa Chata, no. 179, 1990.

———. *Poder, estratificación y salud: Análisis de las condiciones sociales y económicas de la enfermedad en Yucatán.* México DF: Ediciones de la Casa Chata, 1981.

———. "Medicina tradicional, atención primaria y la problemática del alcoholismo." In *Medicina tradicional y atención primaria: Ensayos en homenaje a Gonzalo Aquirre Beltran,* 19–45. México: Cuardernos de la Casa Chata, No. 159, 1987).

———. "Recursos y prácticas médicas 'tradicionales." In *La medicina invisible: Introducción al estudio de la medicina tradicional de México.* Ed. by Xavier Lozoya and Carlos Zolla, 38–61. México DF: Folios Ediciones, 1983.

Merzon, Michael H., Robert E. Black, and Anne J. Mills. "Introduction." *International Public Health: Diseases, Programs, Systems, and Policies.* Ed. by Michael H. Merson, Robert E. Black, and Anne J. Mills, xvii-xxx. Gaithersburg, MD: Aspen Publishers, 2001.

Miles, Ann, and Thomas Leatherman. "Perspectives on Medical Anthropology in the Andes." In Joan D. Koss-Chioino, Thomas Leatherman, and Christine Greenway, 3–15. *Medical Pluralism in the Andes.* New York: Routledge, 2003.

Módena, María Eugenia. *Madres, médicos y curanderos: diferencia cultural e identidad ideológica.* Hidalgo: Ediciones de Casa Chata, 1990.

Montalvo Ortega, Enrique, and Iván Vallado Fajardo. *Yucatán: Sociedad, economía, política, cultura.* México DF: Universidad Nacional Autónoma de México, 1997.

Moreno Cueto, Enrique, Julio Miguel Viveros, Miguel A. Díaz de Sandi, Martha I. García Ugarte, and Eduardo Césarman Vitis. *Sociología Histórica de las Instituciones de Salud.* México DF: IMSS, 1982.

Mullan, Fitzhugh. *Plagues and Politics: The Story of the United States Public Health Service.* New York: Basic Books, 1989.

Muriel, Josefina. *Hospitales de la Nueva España. Tomo II. Fundaciones de los Siglos XVII y XVIII.* México DF: Editorial Jus, 1960.

Nash, June C. *Maya Visions: The Quest for Autonomy in an Age of Globalization.* New York: Routledge, 2001.

Niblo, Stephen R. *Mexico in the 1940s: Modernity, Politics, and Corruption.* Wilmington, DL: Scholarly Resources, 1999.

Nigenda-López, Gustavo. *The Medical Profession, the State and Health Policy in Mexico,* 1917–1988 (D. Phil. London School of Economics and Political Science, 1995).

Novelo Torres, Ernesto. *Discursos al pueblo yucateco.* Mérida: Imprenta Oriente, 1944.

La nueva estructura económica de Yucatán. Consideraciones, documentos y hechos relacionados con la más trascendenta obra de la revolución en materia agraria. Genesis y formación de "Henequeneros de Yucatán." México DF: Editorial "Al Servicio del Pueblo," 1938.

Obregón, Diana. "Building National Medicine: Leprosy and Power in Colombia, 1870–1910." *Social History of Medicine* 15:1 (April 2002): 89–108.

Oliver, Lilia. "El Cólera en los Barrios de Guadalajara." In *Salud, Cultura y Sociedad en América Latina: Nuevas Perspectivas Históricas.* Ed. by Marcos Cueto, 87–109. Lima: IEP y OPS, 1996.

———. "La Pandemia de Cólera Morbos: El Caso de Guadalajara." In *Ensayos Sobre laHistoria de las Epidemias en México.* Vol. 2. Edited by Enrique Florescano and Elsa Malvado, 565–81. México DF: IMSS, 1982.

Omran, Abdel R. "The Epidemiological Transition Theory: A Theory of the Epidemiology of Population Change." *Milbank Memorial Fund Quarterly* 49 (1971): 509–38.

Ortega Canto, Judith. *Henequén y salud*. Mérida: Universidad Autónoma de Yucatán, 1987.

Ortiz de Montellano, Bernard R. *Aztec Medicine, Health, and Nutrition*. New Brunswick: Rutgers University Press, 1990.

Osado, Ricardo, and Dorothy Andrews Heath de Zapata. *El libro del judío, o, Medicina doméstico [i.e. doméstica]: descripción de los nombres de las yerbas de Yucatán y las enfermedades a que se aplican, siglo XVII [i.e.XVIII]*. Mérida: D. Andrews Heath de Zapata, 1979.

Palma Solís, Marco Antonio. *La educación médica en Yucatán*. Mérida: Universidad Autónoma de Yucatán, 1990.

Palma Solís, Marco Antonio, Rubén Salvador Poot Salazar, Rubén Cámara Vallejos. "Antecedentes de la atención primaria de la salud en Yucatán y la Universidad Autónoma de Yucatán." In *Programa UNI-Mérida: una experiencia en la atención primaria de la salud*. Ed. by Marco Antonio Palma Solís, 43–88. Mérida: Ediciones de la Universidad Autónoma de Yucatán, 2003.

Palmer, Steven Paul. "Beginnings of Cuban Bacteriology: Juan Santos Fernández, Medical Research, and the Search for Scientific Sovereignty, 1880–1920." *Hispanic American Historical Review* 91:3 (August 2011): 445–468.

———. *From Popular Medicine to Medical Populism: Doctors, Healers, and Public Power in Costa Rica,* 1800–1940. Durham: Duke University Press, 2003.

———. *Launching Global Health: The Caribbean Odyssey of the Rockefeller Foundation*. Ann Arbor: University of Michigan Press, 2010.

Palmer, Steven and Claudia Agostoni. "Introduction: Landscapes of Latin American Health, 1870–1970." *Canadian Journal of Latin American and Caribbean Studies* 35:69 (2010): 5–18.

Pan American Sanitary Bureau. *Transactions of the Seventh Pan American Sanitary Conference of the American Republics, Held in Havana Cuba, November 5 to 15, 1924*. Washington, DC: PASB, 1924.

Pan American Union. *Transactions of the Fourth International Sanitary Conference of the American Republics, held in Havana, Cuba, November 5 to 15, 1924.* Washington, DC: Pan American Union, 1910.

Pani, Alberto. *Hygiene in Mexico: A Study of Sanitary and Educational Problems*. Trans. by Ernest L. de Gogorza. New York and London: Knickerbocker Press, 1917.

Parra, Pilar Alicia. "Midwives in the Mexican Health System." *Social Science and Medicine* 37:11 (1993): 1321–29.

Pasos Peniche, Manuel. *Historia de la industria henequenero desde 1945 hasta nuestros días*. Mérida: Talleres Gráficas y Editorial "Zamná," 1974.

Patch, Robert. *Maya and Spaniard in Yucatan,* 1648–1812. Stanford: Stanford University Press, 1993.

Peard, Julyan G. *Race, Place, and Medicine: The Idea of the Tropics in Nineteenth Century Brazilian Medicine*. Durham, NC: Duke University Press, 1999.

Pellicer de Brody, Olga, and José Luis Reyes. *Historia de la Revolución Mexicana: Periodo 1952–1960*. No. 22. México DF: El Colegio de México, 1978.

Pio Pérez, Juan C., Hermann Berendt, and Raquel Birman Furman. *Recetarios de indios en lengua maya: índices de plantas medicinales y de enfermedades coordinados por D. Juan Pío Pérez con estractos de los recetarios, notas y añadiduras por C. Hermann Berendt, M.D., Mérida 1870*. México DF: Universidad Nacional Autónoma de México, 1996.

Pérez de Sarmiento, Marisa, and Franco Savarino Roggero. *El cultivo de las élites. Grupos económicos y politicos en Yucatán en los siglos XIX y XX*. México DF: Conaculta, 2001.

Peniche Barrera, Roldán. *Yucatán: Ensayos históricos y literarios*. Mérida: Ediciones de la Universidad Autónoma de Yucatán, 2001.

Plesset, Isabel R., *Noguchi and His Patrons*. Rutherford, NJ: Fairleigh Dickinson University Press, 1980.

Porter, Roy. *The Greatest Benefit to Mankind: A Medical History of Humanity from Antiquity to the Present*. New York: HarperCollins Publishers, 1997.

Power, Helen J. *Tropical Medicine in the Twentieth Century: A History of Liverpool School of Tropical Medicine*. London: Kegan Paul International, 1999.

Press, Irwin. "Problems in the Definition and Classification of Medical Systems." *Social Science and Medicine* 1:14B (1980): 45–57.

———. *Tradition and Adaptation: Life in a Modern Yucatan Maya Village*. Westport, CT: Greenwood Press, 1975.

Prieto I. *The Supreme Board of Health of Mexico: Its History*. México DF: Consejo Superior de Salubridad, 1903.

Puerto, Alexandra. "Henequen Monoculture, Maya Labor, and Infant Mortality in Postrevolutionary Yucatán." In *Women, Ethnicity, and Medical Authority: Historical Perspectives on Reproductive Health in Latin America*. Anne S. Blum, Alexandra Puerto, Tamera Marko, and Adam Warren, 27–49 (Center for Iberian and Latin American Studies. University of California, San Diego). CILAS Working Papers. 2004.

Quevedo, Emilio, Catalina Borda, Juan Carlos Eslava, Claudia Mónica García, María Del Pilar Guzmán, Paola Mejía, and Carlos Ernesto Moguera. *Café y Gusanos, Mosquitos y Petróleo: El Tránsito desde la Higiene hacia la Medicina Tropical y la Salud Pública en Colombia,* 1873–1953. Bogotá: Universidad Nacional de Colombia, Facultad de Medicina, Instituto de Salud Pública, 2004.

Quezada, Noemí. *Enfermedad y Maleficio: El Curandero en el México Colonial.* México D F: UNAM, 1989.

———. "The Inquisition's Repression of *Curanderos*." In *Cultural Encounters: The Impact of the Inquisition in Spain and the New World*. Ed. by Mary Elizabeth Perry and Anne J. Cruz, 39–41. Berkeley: University of California Press, 1991.

Quezada, Sergio. *Breve historia de Yucatán*. México: El Colegio de México, 2001.

Ramírez Carrillo, Luis Alfonso. *Sociedad y población urbana en Yucatán, 1950–1989*. México DF: El Colegio de México, 1993.

Redfield, Robert. *The Folk Culture of Yucatan*. Chicago: University of Chicago Press, 1941.

———. *A Village that Chose Progress: Chan Kom Revisited.* Chicago: University of Chicago Press, 1962.

——— and Alfonso Villa Rojas. *Chan Kom: A Maya Village.* Washington, DC: Carnegie Institution of Washington, publication 448, 1934.

——— and Margaret Park Redfield. "Disease and its Treatment in Dzitas, Yucatán." In *Contributions to American Anthropology and History*, No. 32, 51–81. Washington, DC: Carnegie Institution of Washington, 1940.

Reed, Nelson A. *The Caste War of Yucatán.* Revised edition. Stanford: Stanford University Press, 2001.

Restall Matthew. *The Black Middle Africans, Mayas, and Spaniards in Colonial Yucatán.* Stanford: Stanford University Press, 2009.

———. "The Janus Face of Maya Identity in Post-Conquest Yucatán." In *Maya Survivalism. Acta Mesoamericana*, Vol. 12, 15–23. Verlag: Anton Saurwein, 2001.

———. *The Maya World: Yucatec Culture and Society, 1550–1850.* Stanford: Stanford University Press, 1997.

Risse, Guenter B. "Shelter and Care for Natives and Colonists: Hospitals in Sixteenth-Century New Spain." In *Searching for the Secrets of Nature: The Life and Works of Dr. Francisco Hernández.* Ed. by Simon Varey, Rafael Chabrán, and Dora B. Weiner, 65–81. Stanford: Stanford University Press, 2000.

Rockwell, Elise. "Schools of the Revolution: Enacting and Contesting State Forms in Tlaxcala, 1910–1930." In *Everyday Forms of State Formation: Revolution and the Negotiation of Rule in Modern Mexico.* Ed. by Gilbert M. Joseph and Daniel Nugent, 170–208. Durham: Duke University Press, 1994.

Rodríguez, Martha Eugenia. "Las Juntas de Sanidad en la Nueva España, Siglos XVIII y XIX." *Revista de Investigación Clínica* 53:3 (May–June, 2001): 276–80.

———. "Legislación Sanitaria y Boticas Novohispanas." *Estudios Historicos Novohispanos* 17 (1997): 151–69.

Rodríguez de Romo, Ana Cecilia. "Los Médicos Como Gremio de Poder en el Porfiriato."*Boletín Mexicano de Historia y Filosofía de Medicina* 5:2 (2002): 4–9.

Rodríguez, Julia. *Civilizing Argentina: Science, Medicine, and the Modern State.* Chapel Hill: The University of North Carolina Press, 2006.

Rodríguez, Julia, and Ann Zulawski. "Science and Medicine in Latin America." *Hispanic American Historical Review* (Special Edition: "Science and Medicine in Latin America." Essays in Honor of Nancy Leys Stepan) 91:3 (August 2011): 387–408.

Rojas Aguilar, Gil. "Informe del Delegado Sanitario en Yucatán." In *memoria de la Primera Convención de Fiebre Amarilla, Octubre* 15–20 *de 1921,* 143–46. México DF: DSP, 1921.

Ronzón, José. *Sanidad y modernización en los puertos del Alto Caribe, 1870–1915.* México DF: Universidad Autónoma Metropolitana, 2004.

Rosen, George. *A History of Public Health.* New York: MD Publications, 1958.

Rosenberg, Charles E. *The Cholera Years: The United States in 1832, 1849, and 1866.* Chicago: University of Chicago Press, 1987.

Ross, Paul. *From Sanitary Police to Sanitary Dictatorship: Mexico's Nineteenth-Century Public Health Movement.* (Ph. D. dissertation, University of Chicago, 2005).

———. “Mexico’s Superior Health Council and the American Public Health Association: The Transnational Archive of Porfirian Public Health, 1887–1910.” *Hispanic American Historical Review* 89:4 (November 2009): 573–602.

Roys, Ralph. *The Ethno-Botany of the Maya*. New Orleans: Tulane University, 1931. Republished by ISHI Reprints on Latin America and the Caribbean. Philadelphia, 1976.

———. *The Political Geography of the Yucatán Maya*. Washington, DC: Carnegie Institution of Washington, Publication 613, 1957.

Rugeley, Terry. *Rebellion Now and Forever: Mayas, Hispanics, and Caste War Violence in Yucatán, 1800–1880*. Stanford: Stanford University Press, 2009.

———. *Yucatán’s Maya Peasantry and the Origins of the Caste War*. Austin: University of Texas Press, 1996.

Ruz Quijano, Benito. *Album de recortes de un médico mexicano*. Mérida: Np, 1940.

Sabido Montalvo, Rafael. “Problems asistenciales de los ejidatarios Henequeneros de Yucatán.” In Congreso Médico Peninsular. *Memorias del segundo congreso médico peninsular*. 253–260. Mérida: Díaz Massa, 1945.

Sacristán, Cristiana. “Para integrar a la nación. Terapéutica deportiva y artística en el Manicomio La Castañeda en un momento de reconstrucción nacional, 1920–1940.” In *Estudios de Historia Moderna y Contemporánea de México* 19. Ed. by Claudia Agostini, 99–123. México DF: Universidad Nacional Autónoma de México, 1999.

Sarmiento, Domingo. *Facundo: Civilization and Barbarism*. Trans. by Roberto Eche, Varría González, and Kathleen Ross. Berkeley: University of California Press, 2003.

Sayer, Derek. “Everyday forms of State Formation: Some Dissident Remarks on ‘Hegemony’.” In *Everyday Forms of State Formation: Revolution and the Negotiation of Rule in Modern Mexico*. Ed. by Gilbert M. Joseph and Daniel Nugent, 367–77. Durham: Duke University Press, 1994.

Schackt, Jon. “The Emerging Maya: A Case of Ethnogenesis.” In *Maya Survivalism, Acta Mesoamericana* 12, 3–14. Verlag: Anton Saurwein, 2001.

Schendel, Gordon. *Medicine in Mexico*. Austin: University of Texas Press, 1968.

Schüren, Ute. “Milpa in Crisis”? Changing Agricultural Practices Among Rural Producers in Campeche.” In *Maya Survivalism. Acta Mesoamericana* 12, 263–79. Verlag: Anton Saurwein, 2001.

Seidelin, Harald. “Report of Yellow Fever Expedition to Yucatán, 1911–1912,” *Yellow Fever Bureau Bulletin* 2:2 (October 1912), 123–234.

Shattuck, George Cheever, and Joseph C. Bequaert. *The Peninsula of Yucatan, Medical, Biological, Meteorological and Sociological Studies*. Washington: Carnegie Institution of Washington, 1933.

Siurob, José. “La Sanidad en México.” *Boletín de la Oficina Sanitaria Panamericana* 15:12 (December 1939): 48–53.

———. *Social Medicine in Mexico*. México DF: DSP, 1940.

———. *Trabajo Sanitario en los Estados Unidos Mexicanos, 1934–1940*. México DF: DSP, 1940.

Smith, Frances E. “Medicine in Mexico.” *The Lancet* 208:5373 (1926): 413.

Smith, Stephanie J. *Gender and the Mexican Revolution: Yucatán Women and the Realities of Patriarchy*. Chapel Hill: The University of North Carolina Press, 2009.

Solorzano, Armando. "La Influencia de la Fundación Rockefeller en la Conformación de la Profesión Médica Mexicana, 1921–1949." *Revisita Mexicana de Sociología* 58:1 (1996): 173–203.

———. "The Rockefeller Foundation in Mexico: Nationalism, Public Health and Yellow Fever (1911–1924)" (Ph. D. dissertation, University of Madison, 1990).

———. "The Rockefeller Foundation in Revolutionary Mexico: Yellow Fever in Yucatan and Veracruz." In *Missionaries of Science: The Rockefeller Foundation and Latin America*. Ed. by Marcos Cueto, 52–71. Bloomington: Indiana University Press, 1994.

———. "Sowing the Seeds of Neo-imperialism: The Rockefeller Foundation's Yellow Fever Campaign in Mexico." *International Journal of Health Services* 22 (1992): 529–54.

Somolinos D'Ardois, Germán. *Historia y medicina. Figuras y hechos de la Historiografía médica Mexicana*. México: Imprenta Universitaria, 1957.

Sowell, David. "Multiple Colonizations: State Formation, Public Health and the Yucatec Maya, 1891–1960." In *Crossing Colonial Historiographies: Histories of Colonial and Indigenous Medicines in Transnational Perspective*, eds. Anne Digby, Waltraud Ernst, and Projit B. Muchkarj, 77–97. Cambridge UK: Cambridge Scholars Inc., 2010.

———. *The Tale of Healer Miguel Perdomo Neira: Medicine, Ideologies, and Power in the Nineteenth-Century Andes*. Wilmington, DE: Scholarly Resources, 2001.

———. "Race and the Authorization of Biomedicine in Yucatán, Mexico." In *Health and Medicine in the Circum-Caribbean,* 1800–1968. Ed. by Juanita De Barros, Steven Palmer, and David Wright, 76–97. New York: Routledge Press, 2009.

Stapleton, Darwin H. "Lessons of History? Anti-Malaria Strategies of the International Health Board and the Rockefeller Foundation from the 1920s to the Era of DDT." *Public Health Chronicles* 19 (March-April 2004): 206–15.

Stepan, Nancy. *Beginnings of Brazilian Science: Oswaldo Cruz, Medical Research and Policy,* 1890–1920. New York: Science History Publications, 1981.

Stern, Alexandra Minna. "Yellow Fever Crusade: US Colonialism, Tropical Medicine, and the International Politics of Mosquito Control, 1900–1920." In *Disease, Globalization and Security, 1850 to the Present*. Ed. by Alison Bashford, 41–59. London: Palgrave MacMillan, 2006.

Sullivan, Paul. *Unfinished Conversations: Mayas and Foreigners between Two Wars*. New York: Alfred A. Knopf, 1989.

TePaske, John Jay. "Regulation of Medical Practitioners in the Age of Francisco Hernández." In *Searching for the Secrets of Nature: The Life and Works of Dr. Francisco Hernández*. Ed. by Simon Varey, Rafael Chabrán, and Dora B. Weiner. 55–56. Stanford: Stanford University Press, 2000.

Torre Díaz, Alvaro. *Cuatro años en el Gobierno de Yucatán, 1926–1930*. Mérida: Compañía Tipográfica Yucateca, 1930.

Trask, Benjamin H. *Fearful Ravages. Yellow Fever in New Orleans, 1796–1905*. Lafayette: Center for Louisiana Studies, University of Louisiana at Lafayette, 2005.

Trujillo, Narcisa. "El Maya de las haciendas henequeneras." In *Enciclopedia Yucatanese*. Tomo VI. 133–71. México DF: Edición Oficial del Gobierno de Yucatán, 1977.

Turshen, Meredith. *The Politics of Public Health.* New Brunswick, NJ: Rutgers University Press, 1989.

Urzáiz Jiménez, Carlos. *Crónicas de un estudiante de medicina.* Mérida: Maldonado Editores, 1983.

———. *Desarrollo de las ciencias médicas y la investigación en Yucatán.* Mérida: Talleres Díaz Massa, 1975.

Urzáiz Lares, Enrique. "La arquitectura Porfiriana en Mérida." In *Mérida: El azar y la memoria.* Marco Tulio Peraza Guzmán et. al., 89–114. Mérida: Asociación de Personal Académico, Universidad Autónoma de Yucatán, 1993.

Vargas, Luis Alberto ed., *¿Que debo saber sobre medicina tradicional durante mi servicio social?* México: Editorial del Semenario la Medicina del Hombre en su totalidad, 1981.

Viesca Treviño, Carlos. "Eduardo Liceaga y la Participación Mexicana en la Fundación de la Organización Panamericana de la Salud." *Revista Cubana de Salud Pública* 24:1 (1998): 11–18.

———. "*Curanderismo* in Mexico and Guatemala: Its Historical Evolution from the Sixteenth to the Nineteenth Century." In *Mesoamerican Healers.* Ed. by Brad R. Huber and Alan R. Sandstrom, 37–65. Austin: Texas University Press, 2001.

Villa Rojas, Alfonso. *The Maya of East Central Quintana Roo.* Washington, DC: Carnegie Institution of Washington, 1945.

———. "Terapéutica tradicional y medicina moderna entre los Maya de Yucatán." *Anales de Antropología.* Tomo11. *Etnología y Linguistica,* Vol. XVIII, UNAM (1981): 13–28.

Vivas Arjona, Álvaro, editorial coordinator. *Médicos en Yucatán.* Mérida: Universidad Autónoma de Yucatán, 2010.

Weindling, Paul. "American Foundations and the Internationalizing of Public Health." In *Shifting Boundaries of Public Health: Europe in the Twentieth Century.* Ed. by Susan Gross Soloman, Lion Murard, and Patrick Zylberman, 63–86. Rochester: University of Rochester Press, 2008.

Weisz, George, and Jesse Olsyzkno-Gryn. "The Theory of Epidemiologic Transition: The Origins of a Citation Classic." *Journal of the History of Medicine and the Allied Sciences* 65:3 (July 2010): 287–326.

Wells, Allen. *Yucatán's Gilded Age: Haciendas, Henequen, and International Harvester, 1860–1915.* Albuquerque: University of New Mexico Press, 1985.

———. "Family Elites in a Boom-and-Bust Economy: the Molinas and Peóns of Porfirian Yucatán." *Hispanic American Historical Review* 62: 2 (May 1982): 224–253.

———. and Gilbert M. Joseph. "Modernizing Visions, Chilango Blueprints, and Provincial Growing Pains: Mérida at the Turn of the Century." *Mexican Studies/ Estudios Mexicanos* 8:2 (Summer 1992): 167–215.

——— and Gilbert M. Joseph. *Summer of Discontent, Seasons of Upheaval: Elite Politics and Rural Insurgency in Yucatán,* 1876–1915. Stanford: Stanford University Press, 1996.

Whitfield, Amy, and Howard Waitzkin. "The Vicissitudes of Public Health Policy in the America." *Latin American Research Review* 44:2 (2009): 216–24.

Wilkinson, Lise. "Burgeoning Visions of Global Public Health: The Rockefeller Foundation, the London School of Hygiene and Tropical Medicine, and the 'Hookworm Connection'." *Studies in History and Philosophy of Biological and Biomedical Sciences* 31:3 (2000): 397–407.

Wilkinson, Lise, and Anne Hardy. *Prevention and Cure: The London School of Hygiene and Tropical Medicine.* London: Kegan Paul, 2001.

Williams, Ralph Chester. *The United States Public Health Service, 1798–1950.* Washington, DC: Commissioned Officers Association of the United States Public Health Service, 1951.

Worboys, Michael. "The Emergence of Tropical Medicine: A Study in the Establishment of a Scientific Specialty." In *Perspectives on the Emergence of Scientific-Disciplines.* Ed. by Gerard Lemaine. Roy MacLeod, Michael Mulkay, and Peter Weingart, 75–98. The Hague: Mouton & Co., 1976.

———. "Manson, Ross and colonial medical policy: tropical medicine in London and Liverpool, 1899–1914." In *Disease, Medicine, and Empire: Perspectives on Western Medicine and the Experience of European Expansion.* Ed. by Roy Macleod and Milton Lewis, 21–37. New York: Routledge, 1988.

Yam Sosa, Martha Beatríz, María Teresa Quiñones Vega, José Emilio Pérez Aquilar. *La medicina tradicional entre los henequeneros y maiceros yucatecas*. Mérida: PACMYC-Dirección General de Culturas Populares, 1992.

Young, James Clay. *Medical Choice in a Mexican Village.* New Brunswick, NJ: Rutgers University Press, 1981.

Zulawksi, Ann. "New Trends in Studies of Science and Medicine in Latin America." *Latin American Research Review* 34:3 (1999): 241–51.

———. *Unequal Cures: Public Health and Political Change in Bolivia, 1900–1950.* Durham: Duke University Press, 2007.

Index

About the Author

David Sowell is a Professor of History at Juniata College. Sowell teaches courses on Latin America, International Studies, and the History of Medicine. He has published *The Early Colombian Labor Movement: Artisans and Politics in Bogotá, 1832–1919, The Tale of Healer Miguel Perdomo Neira: Healing, Ideologies, and Power in the Nineteenth-Century Andes,* and numerous articles and book chapters. His work has focused upon the social history of nineteenth-century Colombia, the history of Bogotá, and the history of medicine in Latin America. Sowell is married and has one child.

www.ingramcontent.com/pod-product-compliance
Ingram Content Group UK Ltd.
Pitfield, Milton Keynes, MK11 3LW, UK
UKHW041630031026
15587UKWH00001B/187

9 781498 517348